WILL IT EVER GO AWAY?

STEVEN R FELDMAN, MD
AND VERONICA K
EMMERICH

WILL IT EVER GO AWAY?

Practical Answers to Your Questions About COVID-19

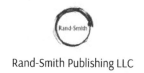

Rand-Smith Publishing LLC

CONTENTS

CONTENTS

Print ISBN: 978-1-950544-26-4
Digital ISBN: 978-1-950544-27-1

First Printing, 2020
Rand-Smith Publishing
www.Rand-Smith.com

Acknowledgements

This book would not have been possible without the guidance of Diane Nine, our agent at Nine Speakers, Inc. We also thank our publishers at Rand-Smith who recognized the importance of this topic and put their trust in us to provide accurate, helpful information to readers. Thank you to the Woolard and Nichols families for their support and encouragement throughout the writing and editing process.

Most of all, we acknowledge and appreciate the many contributors who helped make this book a reality:

Danika Dorelien
Fourth Year Medical Student
New York Medical College
Valhalla, New York
"Travel: Essential and Non-Essential"

Jia C. Gao
Fourth Year Medical Student
New York Medical College
Valhalla, New York
"COVID-19: General Safety"

Erica Ginsburg
Second Year Medical Student
Florida State University College of Medicine

ACKNOWLEDGEMENTS

Tallahassee, Florida
"Exposure to COVID-19, Testing, and Illness"

Shriram Hegde
Clarkstown South High School
West Nyack, New York
"Work, School, and the Office"

Kody Heubach
Second Year Medical Student
Campbell University Jerry M. Wallace School of Osteopathic Medicine
Lillington, North Carolina
"Who is at risk?"

Scott Jaros
Second Year Medical Student
University of North Carolina School of Medicine
Chapel Hill, North Carolina
"Re-opening"
"Sanity"

Rishita Jessu
Fourth Year Medical Student
University of North Texas Health Science Center - Texas College of Osteopathic Medicine
Fort Worth, Texas
"For Healthcare Workers"

Gracie Elena Nguyen
Second Year Medical Student
Kentucky College of Osteopathic Medicine
Pikeville, Kentucky
"A Potential Vaccine"

Adam H. Rosenfeld
Fourth Year Medical Student
University of Missouri School of Medicine

Columbia, Missouri
"Available Treatments"

Lauren Schwartzberg
Fourth Year Medical Student
New York Institute of Technology College of Osteopathic Medicine
Old Westbury, New York
"Avoiding Misinformation"

Aditi Senthilnathan
Fourth Year Medical Student
Wake Forest School of Medicine
Winston-Salem, North Carolina
"Coronavirus: Basics and Background"

CORONAVIRUS: BASICS AND BACKGROUND

What is a coronavirus?

Viruses are tiny infectious particles that can only replicate inside living cells of animals, plants, or bacteria. "Virus" is an umbrella term that encompasses an enormous variety of families and species. These tiny particles, which are not truly considered alive, are responsible for a multitude of human diseases, including measles, polio, and the common cold. They are made of the same genetic material we are made of, called RNA (ribonucleic acid) or DNA (deoxyribonucleic acid), and are surrounded by a protein coat that acts as a protective shell. Some viruses, like coronaviruses, have an additional fatty layer called an envelope. Alcohols, like those found in hand sanitizer, disrupt the protein coat and easily inactivate viruses. Soap dissolves fat and breaks down the fatty coating of enveloped viruses, thereby inactivating them.

Within this vast group of viruses are the coronaviruses. Coronaviruses are a large family of viruses named for the spikes on their surface that resemble a crown. ("Corona" means crown in Latin.) Some coronaviruses cause mild respiratory infections like the common cold, and others cause life-threatening disease. Examples of those that cause dangerous illness are MERS-CoV, which causes Middle East respiratory syndrome, SARS-CoV, which causes severe acute respiratory syndrome[1], and SARS-CoV-2, which causes COVID-19 and is responsible for the current pandemic. The term "SARS-CoV-2" stands for "Severe Acute Respiratory Syndrome-Coronavirus-2." The virus was named this way for its genetic similarity to SARS-CoV, the virus responsible for the SARS outbreak of 2003.

Why is the disease it causes called COVID-19?

"COVID-19" is an abbreviation for the full name of the disease, coronavirus disease 2019, as the outbreak began in 2019. In the abbreviation "CO" stands for corona, "VI" stands for virus, and "D" stands for disease.[2]

How do we know this isn't caused by bacteria?

There have been rumors that COVID-19 is caused by bacteria; these rumors are false. The coronavirus was initially identified in January 2020 by Chinese authorities who took samples from sick patients. They found that the disease had characteristics of a virus, not of bacteria. The Chinese scientists discovered the genetic sequence of this novel virus and then shared it so that other countries could test their sick patients for the same virus. Other countries then began reporting positive cases based on this test.[3] Scientists have also seen the virus (taken from samples of sick patients) under a special type of microscope called an electron microscope, which has an extremely high power, and confirmed that it looks like other coronaviruses.[4]

Where and how did COVID-19 start? What is zoonotic spread?

On December 31, 2019, an outbreak of severe pneumonia cases was reported in the city of Wuhan, China. This was linked to a seafood and animal market in the city. Many of the sick patients worked at or frequently visited this market, and samples taken from the market itself tested positive for SARS-CoV-2. All the current evidence suggests that there was zoonotic spread of the virus, which means that the disease was spread from animals to humans. Based on the genetic sequence of SARS-CoV-2 and its similarity to that of SARS-CoV-1 and other coronaviruses, scientists believe that it also originated in bats. However, it is likely that the disease spread from bat to human through another animal—wild or domestic—rather than directly. It is currently unknown what this animal, called the "intermediate host," is.[5]

How did the novel coronavirus come to the United States?

The first case of COVID-19 in the United States was confirmed on January 20, 2020, in Washington state. The patient, a 35-year-old man who had returned from visiting family in Wuhan, China, on January 14, was tested after he presented to an urgent care center on January 19 with symptoms.[6] Research suggests that the first cases in the United States were in those who had traveled to China; others who had traveled to Europe subsequently contributed to the spread of the disease in the U.S.[7]

What's the difference between an epidemic and a pandemic?

The term "epidemic" refers to a sudden increase in amount of disease above what is expected for a given population. This is limited to a particular geographic area. For example, in the United States, every year in the fall and winter seasons we have an epidemic of the flu. Once an epidemic spreads to other countries and continents, it is called a pandemic. Aside from COVID-19, another example of this is the Swine Flu (H1N1) pandemic of 2009.

How does the virus spread?

COVID-19 is spread via respiratory droplets from person to person. When a person talks, coughs, or sneezes, these tiny droplets can land on another person's nose or mouth. The respiratory droplets can travel up to 6 feet, which is why spread is more likely when people are within 6 feet of one another. These droplets can land on non-living surfaces, where a small amount of virus may remain viable for 4-72 hours. We can unknowingly pick these up with our hands and transfer them to our eyes, nose, and mouth. It is important that we wash our hands throughout the day to reduce the risk of this type of transfer. However, it is thought that the main mode of spread is person-to-person rather than from contact with objects. COVID-19 may also be spread via the airborne route, meaning some droplets can remain suspended in the air and may be inhaled by others even after the infected person is no longer present.[8,9] The extent to which airborne transmission contributes to COVID-19 spread remains unclear. In any case, face masks are an important and effective protective measure.[10]

What is the incubation period?

The incubation period is the length of time between exposure to a disease and initial appearance of symptoms. Half of all people who develop symptoms of COVID-19 will do so within four to five days of exposure, and 99% of people who develop symptoms will do so within 14 days.[11]

What is viral shedding? What are asymptomatic spread and community spread?

Viral shedding refers to the release of virus from an infected individual into the environment. Not all infected individuals have symptoms or know they are infected; they may still shed the virus and contribute to spread of the disease. This is known as asymptomatic spread. Community spread is when people in an area become infected without knowing how or where it happened. This underscores the importance of wearing masks and staying at home when possible.

What are super-spreaders? Are there any documented coronavirus super-spreaders?

The concept of "super-spreaders" is not unique to COVID-19; it refers to an increased tendency to transmit the disease to others. It can be used to describe people, events, or policies. There are data to suggest that a small percent of COVID-19 cases transmit most of the infection.[12] This phenomenon helps explain the variation in infection rates in different groups after exposure to an infected individual. In order to explain the different propagation rates in different countries, one researcher proposed that when super-spreaders infect others, these infected individuals are more likely to become super-spreaders themselves; this may be due to increased viral load in super-spreaders.[13]

There have been documented coronavirus super-spreaders. After a 2.5-hour Skagit County Choir practice in Washington state where one symptomatic person was in attendance, 53 out of 61 people who attended the practice became ill. During the practice, members likely were in close proximity to one another. Singing may have caused more particles to be released because emission increases with increased loudness of voice, and it is thought that some people release more particles when talking than others.[14]

Although evidence for super-spreading exists, one author warns that the term can be problematic in that it is vague and may lead to increased moral blame of certain individuals, which can increase stigma and discourage people from coming forth about recent activities and exposures.[15] In any case, universal use of face masks in public and social distancing reduce the risk of super-spreading events.

What are the symptoms?

Possible symptoms include fever, chills, cough, increased sputum with or without blood, shortness of breath, sore throat, nasal congestion, nausea, vomiting, diarrhea, abdominal pain, loss of appetite, loss of smell or taste, dizziness, confusion, headache, muscle or joint pains, fatigue, and rash. It is not necessary to have all or many of these symptoms to have the disease. The most common symptoms are dry cough, fatigue, and fever. Loss of appetite and diarrhea can also be common and can sometimes be the first symptoms.[16] Additionally, there have been reports that sudden-onset loss of smell in the absence of other symptoms may occur.[17]

What is R_0 and what does it mean for coronavirus?

R_0 (pronounced "R-naught") refers to the basic reproductive number. This is the average number of people that a single person spreads the infection to, assuming no one has immunity to the disease. If the R_0 in a given population is less than 1, it means the spread of the disease will decrease. If the R_0 is 1, it means that on average each infected person spreads the disease to one more person—so the rate of disease will be stable and will not cause an outbreak. If the R_0 is greater than 1, an epidemic may occur. One estimate suggests that the R_0 for COVID-19 is between 2 and 3.5 at the early stage (which is higher than that of SARS or MERS)[18]; a more recent estimate suggests that it may be as high as 5.7.[19] In order to stop transmission of the disease, interventions such as social distancing and vaccination to produce immunity are important. The higher the R_0, the more intervention efforts are necessary to control the spread of the virus.

What is the mortality rate? Is this different from the case-fatality ratio?

The mortality rate is number of deaths divided by the total number of cases. One estimate of the mortality rate for COVID-19 is 2.6%.[20] This is difficult to determine exactly because we do not know the total number of cases or deaths. As testing is typically done only on symptomatic individuals who seek testing, the number of confirmed cases that we know of is likely an underestimate of the true prevalence. There are also many deaths that are never confirmed to be the result of COVID-19. This is why case-fatality ratios can be helpful.

The **observed** case-fatality ratio is the number of deaths per 100 confirmed cases. In the United States, the observed case-fatality ratio is 5.8%.[21] On the other hand, the **symptomatic** case-fatality ratio is the number of symptomatic individuals who die from disease out of all symptomatic infected individuals. An individual does not need to have a confirmed case of COVID-19 to be included in the symptomatic case-fatality ratio; he or she is presumed to have COVID-19 based on symptoms and a suggestive history. An estimate of the symptomatic case-fatality ratio in the United States is 0.4%.[22] Many symptomatic individuals do not undergo testing, so the denominator for the symptomatic case-fatality ratio is likely larger than that of the observed case-fatality ratio.

Is the influenza vaccine protective against COVID-19? How about the pneumonia vaccine?

No, but these vaccines may still be helpful. The flu shot is effective against the influenza virus but is not effective against COVID-19. The pneumonia vaccine helps protect from bacterial pneumonia but not against COVID-19. However, being infected simultaneously with both SARS-CoV-2 and the flu or bacterial pneumonia can increase the risk for severe disease, especially in older adults. In older or at-risk adults who can safely obtain these vaccines, they may help decrease morbidity and mortality associated with COVID-19.[23] A yearly flu shot is recommended for everyone.

How does COVID-19 compare to the flu? To SARS?

COVID-19, the flu, and SARS are all caused by viruses that can affect the respiratory tract. Both COVID-19 and the flu can cause similar symptoms, and both can cause pneumonia.

The incubation period, or time between becoming infected to showing symptoms, is shorter for the flu (1-2 days) than for COVID-19 (4-6 days).[24] Although the flu infects more people than COVID-19, COVID-19 has a higher mortality rate and can cause more severe disease. The mortality rate for the flu is 0.07%-0.2%; the mortality rate of COVID-19 has been estimated to be 2.6%. The flu is also less infectious than COVID-19. The R_0 for the flu ranges from 0.9 to 2.1, which is lower than that of COVID-19 (between 2 and 3.5).[20,25]

Both SARS (caused by SARS-CoV) and COVID-19 (caused by SARS-CoV-2) are due to coronaviruses, and they are both thought to have originated in bats. SARS was originally reported in China in 2003, and also caused severe respiratory illness with symptoms like those of COVID-19. The incubation period for SARS is around five days, similar to that of COVID-19. SARS-CoV caused 8,422 cases of SARS worldwide and 919 deaths, and the pandemic resolved by the end of that year. In contrast, by February 2020 there were 72,436 confirmed cases of COVID-19 in China alone and 1,868 deaths. The estimated mortality rate of COVID-19 is lower than that of SARS (which has a mortality rate of 11%) but there are many more cases of COVID-19 than there were of SARS. The estimated R_0 of SARS is 2 to 4, similar to that of COVID-19.[20,26] The fact that COVID-19 has a lower mortality rate than SARS may explain why there are so many more cases of COVID-19 despite both having a similar R_0. Many individuals with mild or asymptomatic COVID-19 are unaware of their diagnosis; isolation and containment are thus not possible, and the likelihood of spread is increased.

Can I get COVID-19 from my pet or another animal?

Although the original source of the virus is thought to have been an animal, there is no evidence currently to suggest that pets can cause COVID-19 in humans. There is a small risk of transmitting COVID-19 from humans to pets, so social distancing rules apply to non-human members of a household as well. There is currently no recommendation for pets to wear face masks; they may not be effective. The disease is generally mild in animals if they do become infected.[27,28]

Can I get COVID-19 from ticks or mosquitoes?

There is currently no evidence to suggest that COVID-19 can be spread by ticks or mosquitos.[29]

Will COVID-19 die down in warmer weather (i.e., summer)?

We do not know if COVID-19 will die down in the summer. Countries in the Southern Hemisphere, like Brazil and Australia, experienced the start of the pandemic during their summer months. As of June 29, 2020, Brazil had the second highest number of cumulative cases in the world.[30] A recent study conducted in Australia found that low humidity was associated with higher rates of COVID-19, but found no relationship between temperature and disease rates.[31] Although climate can affect the seasonality of endemic diseases like the flu, researchers believe that higher summertime temperatures will not be enough to limit the spread of COVID-19 and that severe outbreaks will still occur.[32]

What is the risk of a second (or third) wave?

Many experts believe there will be an increase in cases in the fall and that there may even be a third wave after that. An increase in cases in the fall may coincide with the start of the flu season, which may pose unique challenges in terms of distinguishing between the two illnesses. However, knowing that this will likely occur may provide us an opportunity to better prepare.[33]

Will COVID-19 become seasonal, similar to the flu? Why are some viruses seasonal?

It is possible that COVID-19 may eventually express seasonality like the flu, with more cases occurring in the winter months. It is thought that some viruses like the flu are seasonal in regions with winter months because the virus can survive longer in cold, dry air.

However, early in the stages of a pandemic, nobody has immunity and viruses spread rapidly because everyone is susceptible. It is only later, when many people have been infected and have some amount of immunity, that a virus shows sensitivity to seasonal influences. At this point, because SARS-CoV-2 is a new virus and because people are not immune to it, it will likely not be confined to particular seasons.[34]

References

1. Fehr AR, Perlman S. Coronaviruses: an overview of their replication and pathogenesis. *Methods in molecular biology (Clifton, NJ).* 2015;1282:1-23.
2. Centers for Disease Control and Prevention. Coronavirus Disease 2019 Basics. https://www.cdc.gov/coronavirus/2019-ncov/faq.html. Updated June 2, 2020. Accessed June 5, 2020

3. World Health Organization. Novel Coronavirus (2019-nCoV) Situation Report – 1 21 January 2020. https://www.who.int/docs/default-source/coronaviruse/situation-reports/20200121-sitrep-1-2019-ncov.pdf?sfvrsn=20a99c10_4. Published January 20, 2020. Accessed June 5, 2020.

4. Kim J-M, Chung Y-S, Jo HJ, et al. Identification of Coronavirus Isolated from a Patient in Korea with COVID-19. *Osong Public Health Res Perspect.* 2020;11(1):3-7.

5. World Health Organization. Coronavirus disease 2019 (COVID-19) Situation Report – 94. https://www.who.int/docs/default-source/coronaviruse/situation-reports/20200423-sitrep-94-covid-19.pdf. Published April 23, 2020. Accessed June 5, 2020.

6. Holshue ML, DeBolt C, Lindquist S, et al. First Case of 2019 novel coronavirus in the United States. *New England Journal of Medicine.* 2020;382(10):929-936.

7. Centers for Disease Control and Prevention. Evidence for limited early spread of COVID-19 within the United States, January—February 2020. https://www.cdc.gov/mmwr/volumes/69/wr/mm6922e1.htm. Published May 29, 2020. Accessed June 5, 2020.

8. Lotfi M, Hamblin MR, Rezaei N. COVID-19: Transmission, prevention, and potential therapeutic opportunities [published online ahead of print, 2020 May 29]. *Clin Chim Acta.* 2020; 508:254–266.

9. Leung NHL, Chu DKW, Shiu EYC, et al. Respiratory virus shedding in exhaled breath and efficacy of face masks. *Nature Medicine.* 2020;26(5):676-680.

10. Zhang R, Li Y, Zhang AL, Wang Y, Molina MJ. Identifying airborne transmission as the dominant route for the spread of COVID-19. *Proceedings of the National Academy of Sciences.* 2020;117(26):14857-14863.

11. The incubation period of coronavirus disease 2019 (COVID-19) from publicly reported confirmed cases: estimation and application. *Annals of Internal Medicine.* 2020;172(9):577-582.

12. Kenyon C. The prominence of asymptomatic super-spreaders in transmission mean universal face masking should be part of COVID-19 de-escalation strategies. *Int J Infect Dis.* 2020: S1201-9712(1220)30409-30404.

13. Beldomenico PM. Do superspreaders generate new superspreaders? A hypothesis to explain the propagation pattern of COVID-19. *Int J Infect Dis.* 2020; 96:461-463.

14. Hamner L, Dubbel P, Capron I, et al. High SARS-CoV-2 Attack rate following exposure at a choir practice - Skagit County, Washington, March 2020. *MMWR Morbidity and mortality weekly report.* 2020;69(19):606-610.

15. Cave E. COVID-19 Super-spreaders: definitional quandaries and implications. *Asian Bioeth Rev.* 2020:1-8.

16. Gulati A, Pomeranz C, Qamar Z, et al. A comprehensive review of manifestations of novel coronaviruses

in the context of deadly COVID-19 global pandemic. *Am J Med Sci.* 2020.

17. Gane SB, Kelly C, Hopkins C. Isolated sudden onset anosmia in COVID-19 infection. A novel syndrome? *Rhinology.* 2020;58(3):299-301.

18. Wang Y, Wang Y, Chen Y, Qin Q. Unique epidemiological and clinical features of the emerging 2019 novel coronavirus pneumonia (COVID-19) implicate special control measures. *J Med Virol.* 2020:10.1002/jmv.25748.

19. Sanche S, Lin YT, Xu C, Romero-Severson E, Hengartner N, Ke R. High Contagiousness and rapid spread of severe acute respiratory syndrome coronavirus 2. *Emerging infectious diseases.* 2020;26(7).

20. Yang Y, Peng F, Wang R, et al. The deadly coronaviruses: The 2003 SARS pandemic and the 2020 novel coronavirus epidemic in China. J Autoimmun. 2020; 109:102434-102434.

21. Johns Hopkins University Coronavirus Resource Center. Maps and Trends: Mortality Analysis. https://coronavirus.jhu.edu/data/mortality. Updated June 6, 2020. Accessed June 6, 2020.

22. Centers for Disease Control and Prevention. Covid-19 pandemic planning scenarios. https://www.cdc.gov/coronavirus/2019-ncov/hcp/planning-scenarios.html. Updated May 20, 20. Accessed June 6, 2020.

23. Centre for Mathematical Modelling of Infectious Diseases. Use of seasonal influenza and pneumococcal polysaccharide vaccines in older adults to reduce COVID-19 mortality. https://cmmid.github.io/topics/

covid19/covid19_siv_ppv23.html. Published April 25, 2020. Accessed June 6, 2020.

24. Subbarao K, Mahanty S. Respiratory Virus Infections: Understanding COVID-19. *Immunity.* 2020: S1074-7613(1020)30212-30210.

25. Biggerstaff M, Cauchemez S, Reed C, Gambhir M, Finelli L. Estimates of the reproduction number for seasonal, pandemic, and zoonotic influenza: a systematic review of the literature. BMC infectious diseases. 2014; 14:480.

26. World Health Organization. Consensus document on the epidemiology of severe acute respiratory syndrome (SARS). https://www.who.int/csr/sars/en/WHO-consensus.pdf?ua=1. Published May 2003. Accessed June 10, 2020.

27. Oregon Veterinary Medical Association. COVID-19: Coronavirus & Pets FAQ. https://www.oregonvma.org/care-health/zoonotic-diseases/coronavirus-faq. Updated June 3, 2020. Accessed June 6, 2020.

28. Centers for Disease Control and Prevention. Coronavirus Disease 2019 (COVID-19): Pets & Other Animals. https://www.cdc.gov/coronavirus/2019-ncov/daily-life-coping/pets.html. Updated June 2, 2020. Accessed June 6, 2020.

29. Eslami H, Jalili M. The role of environmental factors to transmission of SARS-CoV-2 (COVID-19). *AMB Express.* 2020;10(1):92.

30. Johns Hopkins University Coronavirus Resource Center. Maps and Trends: Cumulative Cases. https://coro-

navirus.jhu.edu/data/cumulative-cases. Updated July 2, 2020. Accessed July 2, 2020.

31. Ward MP, Xiao S, Zhang Z. The role of climate during the COVID-19 epidemic in New South Wales, Australia. *Transboundary and emerging diseases.* 2020.

32. Baker RE, Yang W, Vecchi GA, Metcalf CJE, Grenfell BT. Susceptible supply limits the role of climate in the early SARS-CoV-2 pandemic. *Science (New York, NY).* 2020.

33. Strazewski L. Harvard epidemiologist: Beware COVID-19's second wave this fall. American Medical Association. https://www.ama-assn.org/delivering-care/public-health/harvard-epidemiologist-beware-covid-19-s-second-wave-fall. Published May 8, 2020. Accessed June 6, 2020.

34. Lipsitch M. Seasonality of SARS-CoV-2: Will COVID-19 go away on its own in warmer weather? Center for Communicable Disease Dynamics, Harvard T.H. Chan School of Public Health. https://ccdd.hsph.harvard.edu/will-covid-19-go-away-on-its-own-in-warmer-weather/. Accessed June 6, 2020.

COVID-19: GENERAL SAFETY

What is the best way to protect myself from COVID-19?

The best way to protect yourself is to prevent potential exposure to SARS-CoV-2, the virus that causes COVID-19, in the first place. This virus generally spreads through close contact from person to person by way of respiratory droplets. Close contact is defined as being within 6 feet of someone for at least 15 minutes.[1] Respiratory droplets are often invisible to the naked eye and are produced whenever a person coughs, sneezes, laughs, or speaks. These droplets carry the infectious virus and can land on people or things around you, or they can be breathed in by others.

Since SARS-CoV-2 can be spread by people who are feeling well and asymptomatic,[2] it is important to limit any possible exposure by maintaining a distance of at least 6 feet apart from anyone outside of your household and wearing face coverings whenever you leave your home or when social distancing is not possible. There is evidence that SARS-CoV-2 can survive on some surfaces and objects,[3] so it may be prudent to practice proper and frequent handwashing and to routinely clean and disinfect high-touch surfaces, such as phones, doorknobs, handles, and light switches.

What is the right way to wash my hands?

Proper and frequent handwashing is one of the most effective ways to protect yourself and your community from many types of illnesses and infections,[4,5] including COVID-19. Follow these five steps to properly wash your hands:

1. Wet your hands with clean, running water and apply soap.
2. Lather the soap in your hands by rubbing them together, making sure to rub between your fingers, under fingernails, and the backs and palms of both hands.
3. Keep rubbing your hands for 20 seconds, or the duration of the "Happy Birthday" song two times.[6]
4. Rinse off the soap under clean, running water.
5. Dry your hands with a clean towel or air dryer.

If soap and running water are not readily available, you can use alcohol-based hand sanitizer that contains at least 60% alcohol according to the product label.[7,8] Make sure to dispense enough hand sanitizer to thoroughly wet your hands with the product and rub your hands together until the hand sanitizer evaporates.

Is it better to use soap and water or hand sanitizer?

It is generally better to use soap and water when it is available for a number of reasons. First, hand sanitizers are not effective at cleansing visibly soiled or greasy hands.[9] They are effective at killing most microbes, but cannot physically remove dirt. Next, hand sanitizers do not target all types of germs, and they may not remove other contaminants like chemicals and heavy metals.[10] Lastly, repeated applications of hand sanitizer without a soap and water cleanse in between can lead to product buildup and an uncomfortable film left on the hands.

Does the water temperature matter when I wash my hands?

No, it is fine to use either warm or cold running water to wash your hands; there is no need to use uncomfortably hot water. Water temperature does not have a major effect on germ removal; too hot water can increase skin irritation.[11,12]

How can I minimize skin irritation and dryness from frequent handwashing?

Use a comfortable water temperature that is neither too hot nor too cold, and make sure to thoroughly rinse off any soap when washing your hands (including from the web spaces between the fingers). Using a hand lotion or moisturizer immediately after washing your hands each time may help create a protective barrier and prevent skin dryness and irritation.[13]

What is social distancing and how do I do it properly?

Social distancing refers to physically distancing yourself from other people who do not live with you. To properly social distance, keep at least 6 feet away from other people, do not gather in groups, and avoid crowds. If possible, work from home, and limit your essential errand runs. Maintaining a 6-foot distance can be difficult, but it is especially important if you are living in close quarters, if you or one of your household members is a vulnerable individual, or if you are living in a multi-residence building.

The 6-foot recommendation is based on currently available data about SARS-CoV-2 and its spread. As scientists learn more about the virus, this recommendation may change, reflecting the rapidly growing body of knowledge about SARS-CoV-2.

Are the rules different for social distancing outdoors? Can I go for a run?

Yes, it is safe to exercise outdoors, but if you will be around other people it is recommended to wear a mask or face covering and maintain social distancing of at least 6 feet whenever possible. Vigorous breathing, such as breathing during exercise, can increase the distance that respiratory droplets travel.[14] If you find it difficult to wear a mask during exercise, you may temporarily remove it when you are physically distant from other people.

Although there is some evidence that SARS-CoV-2 is less transmissible in outdoor settings compared with indoor settings, this is highly dependent on various factors such as air temperature, humidity, and sunlight. Sunlight can potentially inactivate the SARS-CoV-2 virus on outdoor surfaces, but since the intensity and duration of sunlight vary depending on time and location, it cannot be relied upon for preventing outdoor transmission.[15,16]

Does social distancing work?

Yes, social distancing dramatically reduces person-to-person transmission of COVID-19.[17-19] Based on simulation studies and recent data from the current pandemic, implementing social distancing measures can lower new infection rates.

One study of 26 countries over a span of five weeks during the pandemic showed that government enforcement of social distancing policies, such as travel and public space restrictions, accounted for around 47% of the variation in COVID-19 transmission rate.[17] Another study in the United Kingdom discovered that social distancing interventions led to a 74% reduction in the average number of daily physical contacts, which is significant enough to reduce the R_0 from 2.6 to 0.62.[19] Based on information from countries around the world, social distancing is very effective at keeping us healthy and preventing our local healthcare systems from becoming overwhelmed with COVID-19 patients.

Should I wear a mask? If so, what kind?

Masks and cloth face coverings are recommended for all children and adults when outside or in places where social distancing is not possible. Do not place masks or face coverings on children under two years old, anyone with breathing difficulties, or anyone who is unable to remove a mask on their own.

Surgical masks and N95 respirator masks are not recommended for use among the general public, as these supplies are still lacking for healthcare professionals who are in close contact with COVID-19 patients. Commercially available facepiece filtering respirators (FFR) with a one-way exhalation valve on the exterior of the mask are also not recommended. This type of mask provides inward protection to the wearer but does not reduce outward spread of infectious particles due to the added exhalation valve. Masks with valves are not recommended for the general public, as they do not adequately prevent COVID-19 transmission.[20,21]

Cloth face coverings can be made from common household items, such as bandanas, scarves, bed sheets, fabric scraps, and other apparel items. Non-stretch, tightly woven, and opaque fabrics are preferred to stretchy, knit, or sheer fabrics, and multiple layers of fabric can be stacked together to increase filtration of respiratory droplets.[22]

Why did experts first recommend not wearing a mask if wearing a mask is so helpful? If they change their minds, why should I believe them?

During the earlier stages of the COVID-19 pandemic, experts initially recommended that only those with symptoms of respiratory illness or caring for patients should wear face masks. This was based on the sparse available data at the time which did not demonstrate a benefit for asymptomatic people to wear face masks. The initial recommendations were also influenced by the global shortage of face masks and other personal protective equipment (PPE) for healthcare workers.

In April 2020, the Centers for Disease Control and Prevention (CDC) updated its guidance to recommend that the general public wear face coverings or masks due to new studies demonstrating SARS-CoV-2 transmission by asymptomatic patients.[2] These changing recommendations reflect the evolving body of knowledge about COVID-19 as researchers around the world share their scientific findings. While there is some uncertainty about other aspects of COVID-19, there is an abundance of evidence showing the importance of wearing masks among the general public to reduce the transmission of COVID-19.

What materials are best for homemade masks?

The two main methods by which face coverings reduce transmission of COVID-19 are through mechanical and electrostatic filtration. Mechanical filtration refers to a material's ability to physically block relatively larger respiratory droplets. Non-porous fabrics with a tight weave, like high thread count cotton sheets or quilting cotton, are best for mechanical filtering of respiratory droplets.

Electrostatic filtration refers to the ability of a material with static charge to attract and trap relatively smaller respiratory droplets. Materials like silk, flannel, and polyester chiffon offer decent electrostatic filtration. A face covering that combines both methods of filtration with two or more layers of fabric offers increased filtration efficiency beyond that offered by mechanical or electrostatic filtration alone.[22,23]

How do I properly wear a mask?

The proper way to wear a mask or face covering is to make sure your nose and mouth are both fully covered, with the top of the mask across the bridge of your nose and the bottom of the mask underneath your chin. Secure the ear loops or ties tightly so that there are as few gaps along the perimeter of the mask and your face as possible. Do not pull and lower your mask to rest underneath your chin, do not leave your nose or mouth exposed, and try not to touch the mask while you are wearing it to avoid accidental contamination.

If you have facial hair, being clean-shaven will create a better seal around your face covering or mask, which may help further reduce spread of respiratory droplets.[24]

What are some wrong ways to wear a mask?

The New York Times has illustrated several ways not to wear a mask, including: wearing the mask below your nose or just covering the tip of your nose, leaving your chin exposed, wearing the mask loosely with gaps on the sides, and pushing your mask under your chin.[25] Wearing a mask incorrectly will allow your breath—and potentially infectious respiratory droplets—to disperse easily around the edges of the mask, defeating much of its purpose.

The simple act of breathing—as well as talking, coughing, and sneezing—generates respiratory droplets and can spread infectious particles from both your nose and mouth. Therefore, wearing a mask under the nose or only covering the tip of the nose largely defeats its purpose. This is why surgeons, anesthesiologists, and nurses who work in operating rooms are required to fully cover their nose and mouth while at work.

Masks are irritating. How can I make them more comfortable to wear?

Face masks can be uncomfortable to wear, but it is important to not touch or adjust your face mask to prevent accidental transmission of germs to your eyes, nose, or mouth. There are a few ways to make face masks and coverings more comfortable so that they can better serve their purpose.

Masks are generally available in two varieties, one with ear loops and another which is secured around the back of the head. If your ears are irritated by contact with the elastic straps, try switching to masks that are secured around your head instead.[26] Alternatively, you can purchase or fashion your own ear loop extenders, which function to hold both ear loops in a position around the back of the head and relieve pressure on the ears.

Commercially available face masks and even some cloth face coverings are made with many different materials and chemicals,[27] some of which may cause skin irritation with prolonged contact. Try applying a layer of moisturizer or petroleum jelly to the areas of your face in contact with the mask prior to putting it on to create a protective barrier.[28,29] In addition to applying a lotion or cream barrier between your skin and the mask, consider changing your mask or fabric. Contact your doctor if skin irritation persists or worsens.

Does the virus survive on surfaces? How long can it survive outside of a host?

SARS-CoV-2 can survive on some surfaces for up to nine days, depending on a variety of factors including the type of surface, environmental temperature, and humidity. The virus appears to survive longer on smooth, non-porous surfaces like glass, steel, and plastic compared with wood and cardboard. However, the virus can be killed with heat, soap and water, and many readily available disinfectants.[30,31] Visit the Environmental Protection Agency website (www.epa.gov/pesticide-registration/list-n-disinfectants-use-against-sars-cov-2-covid-19) for a list of products you can purchase that are effective against SARS-CoV-2.

Although SARS-CoV-2 has been detected on some surfaces, there are no documented cases of COVID-19 transmission from surfaces alone.

Does SARS-CoV-2 survive on clothing? Should I do laundry a certain way?

It is uncertain precisely how long SARS-CoV-2 can survive on clothing and other apparel items, but some studies have found the virus is capable of surviving on clothing for up to two days. The virus is very susceptible to heat and humidity, but it is still recommended to take special precautions if you are ill or living with someone who is ill.[30]

If you and everyone in your household is healthy, the World Health Organization (WHO) recommends laundering your clothes as you normally would, using detergent.[32] If you are washing clothes at a public laundromat or communal laundry room, minimize your time in public spaces and fold your clothes at home.

If you or someone in your household is ill with suspected or confirmed COVID-19, the CDC and WHO recommend taking the following steps to wash and disinfect clothing and linens:

1. Wash the patient's clothes and other linens separately.
2. Use a common household laundry detergent, and make sure to read and follow the product label instructions and the garment care labels to avoid damage to your clothes.
3. Wear gloves when handling any laundry soiled with bodily fluids.
4. Wash clothes on the warmest water setting (between 140°F and 194°F) that is appropriate for your garments and dry clothes thoroughly.[33,34]

Is it safe to order takeout?

Yes, enjoy! COVID-19 transmission has not been reported through food, food packaging, and food preparation. Although there is evidence that the virus can remain on certain surfaces for up to a few days, the best way to stay safe when ordering food from restaurants is to practice social distancing and hand hygiene by requesting contactless delivery and washing your hands after removing any packaging.

How far can the virus travel in the air?

There are many factors that determine how far SARS-CoV-2 can travel in the air. In laboratory environments optimized for maximizing the spread of respiratory droplets, viral particles were able to travel as far as 8-10 meters, or approximately 26-32 feet in the air[14,18]. In these studies, environmental temperature, humidity, wind speed, and wind direction favorable for SARS-CoV-2 dispersion were used to model the distance and trajectory of artificially generated respiratory droplets produced when masks and face coverings are not worn.

However, it is unlikely to encounter the ideal conditions that can reproduce the maximum distance that SARS-CoV-2 can spread in reality, and 6 feet is a safe distance for preventing transmission if everyone is wearing a mask or face covering.

If I have been in isolation for some number of days, is it safe for me to see someone else who has also been in isolation?

While any close contact with someone outside of your household is a risk, it is important for our mental health and emotional well-being to maintain connections with friends and family. Staying at home and remaining in isolation are the lowest risk, but the benefits of being social cannot be entirely overlooked. If you have been responsibly isolating and you trust that the other party has been doing the same, consider harm reduction strategies that lower the risk of spreading or contracting the virus.[35] Aim for smaller group gatherings in large outdoor or well-ventilated spaces where everyone can still practice social distancing. Avoid sharing food or utensils, wash your hands often, and wear your mask or face covering whenever possible. Make sure that everyone attending your social gathering is aware of and agrees to adhere to these safety measures to minimize the risk of COVID-19 transmission.

Is it safe for me to see the doctor for other medical conditions?

If you are not feeling well, you should seek out medical care. In addition, you should continue to see your doctor for management of chronic conditions like hypertension, diabetes, heart disease, and autoimmune diseases. Unless it is an emergency, there are many ways to get in contact with a doctor without leaving your home. Call your doctor's office before visiting in person, as many offices no longer have waiting rooms, some offices may be closed or have modified hours, and others may be able to offer telemedicine consults via phone or video call. If you need to see a doctor in person, make sure to wear a mask or face covering at all times and practice social distancing whenever it is possible.

Is it safe to eat raw fruits and vegetables? Should I wipe my groceries down?

Yes, it is still safe to consume raw fruits and vegetables. It is not necessary to wash or wipe your food with soap or disinfectants. Practice safe food handling as usual and maintain frequent and proper handling before, during, and after food preparation.[36]

Can I catch COVID-19 from the mail and/or packages?

Although the virus can temporarily survive on some surfaces, it is unlikely to be spread by handling mail and packages, especially if you practice safe handling. After receiving mail, packages, or other deliveries, wash your hands with soap and water for 20 seconds or use hand sanitizer containing at least 60% alcohol to disinfect your hands. There are no known cases of COVID-19 transmission occurring via mail or packages.

Should I change my shopping habits?

It is important to go shopping only for necessities like groceries and other essential household items during this time. If you are able, consider ordering groceries and household items for home delivery or curbside pickup. Make larger but less frequent shopping trips to reduce the number of exposures and create a shopping list before you go to limit your time in the stores. Remember to stay at least 6 feet from others while shopping and waiting in lines, wear a mask or face covering at all times, and do not touch your eyes, nose, or mouth. If available, wipe down your shopping cart or basket with disinfecting wipes. Minimize your contact with items and fixtures in the store and use touchless payment methods if possible. Lastly, do not go shopping if you are sick or feeling unwell.

Can I get COVID-19 from drinking water?

No. SARS-CoV-2 viral particles have not been detected in drinking water supplies, and there are no known transmissions of COVID-19 through drinking water contamination.[37]

Can I get COVID-19 from the feces of an infected person?

SARS-CoV-2 has been detected in the feces of some COVID-19 positive patients, but there are no confirmed cases of transmission from the feces of an infected person to another person.[38] Regardless, it is best to be cautious. To prevent accidental fecal-oral transmission, make sure to wash your hands after using the restroom, before food preparation or consumption, and regularly disinfect frequently touched surfaces in your home.

References

1. Zhang N, Su B, Chan PT, Miao T, Wang P, Li Y. Infection spread and high-resolution detection of close contact behaviors. *Int J Environ Res Public Health.* 2020;17(4).
2. Rothe C, Schunk M, Sothmann P, et al. Transmission of 2019-nCoV infection from an asymptomatic contact in Germany. *N Engl J Med.* 2020;382(10):970-971.
3. Kampf G, Todt D, Pfaender S, Steinmann E. Persistence of coronaviruses on inanimate surfaces and their inactivation with biocidal agents. *J Hosp Infect.* 2020;104(3):246-251.

4. Rabie T, Curtis V. Handwashing and risk of respiratory infections: a quantitative systematic review. *Trop Med Int Health.* 2006;11(3):258-267.

5. Aiello AE, Coulborn RM, Perez V, Larson EL. Effect of hand hygiene on infectious disease risk in the community setting: a meta-analysis. *Am J Public Health.* 2008;98(8):1372-1381.

6. Thampi N, Longtin Y, Peters A, Pittet D, Overy K. It's in our hands: a rapid, international initiative to translate a hand hygiene song during the COVID-19 pandemic. *J Hosp Infect.* 2020.

7. Hubner NO, Hubner C, Wodny M, Kampf G, Kramer A. Effectiveness of alcohol-based hand disinfectants in a public administration: impact on health and work performance related to acute respiratory symptoms and diarrhoea. *BMC Infect Dis.* 2010;10:250.

8. Kampf G, Kramer A. Epidemiologic background of hand hygiene and evaluation of the most important agents for scrubs and rubs. *Clin Microbiol Rev.* 2004;17(4):863-893.

9. Pickering AJ, Davis J, Boehm AB. Efficacy of alcohol-based hand sanitizer on hands soiled with dirt and cooking oil. *J Water Health.* 2011;9(3):429-433.

10. Pickering AJ, Boehm AB, Mwanjali M, Davis J. Efficacy of waterless hand hygiene compared with handwashing with soap: a field study in Dar es Salaam, Tanzania. *Am J Trop Med Hyg.* 2010;82(2):270-278.

11. Carrico AR, Spoden M, Wallston KA, Vandenbergh MP. The environmental cost of misinformation: Why the recommendation to use elevated temperatures for

handwashing is problematic. *Int J Consum Stud.* 2013;37(4):433-441.

12. Laestadius JG, Dimberg L. Hot water for handwashing--where is the proof?. *J Occup Environ Med.* 2005;47(4):434-435.

13. Singh M, Pawar M, Bothra A, Choudhary N. Overzealous hand hygiene during the COVID 19 pandemic causing an increased incidence of hand eczema among general population. *J Am Acad Dermatol.* 2020;83(1):e37-e41.

14. Feng Y, Marchal T, Sperry T, Yi H. Influence of wind and relative humidity on the social distancing effectiveness to prevent COVID-19 airborne transmission: A numerical study. *J Aerosol Sci.* 2020:105585.

15. Ratnesar-Shumate S, Williams G, Green B, et al. Simulated Sunlight Rapidly Inactivates SARS-CoV-2 on Surfaces. J Infect Dis. 2020;222(2):214-222.

16. Sagripanti JL, Lytle CD. Estimated inactivation of coronaviruses by solar radiation with special reference to COVID-19. *Photochem Photobiol.* 2020.

17. Delen D, Eryarsoy E, Davazdahemami B. No place like home: Cross-national data analysis of the efficacy of social distancing during the COVID-19 pandemic. *JMIR Public Health Surveill.* 2020;6(2):e19862.

18. Setti L, Passarini F, De Gennaro G, et al. Airborne transmission route of COVID-19: Why 2 meters/6 feet of inter-personal distance could not be enough. *Int J Environ Res Public Health.* 2020;17(8).

19. Jarvis CI, Van Zandvoort K, Gimma A, et al. Quantifying the impact of physical distance measures on the

transmission of COVID-19 in the UK. *BMC Med.* 2020;18(1):124.

20. Kuo YM, Lai CY, Chen CC, Lu BH, Huang SH, Chen CW. Evaluation of exhalation valves. *Ann Occup Hyg.* 2005;49(7):563-568.

21. Ippolito M, Iozzo P, Gregoretti C, Grasselli G, Cortegiani A. Facepiece filtering respirators with exhalation valve should not be used in the community to limit SARS-CoV-2 diffusion. *Infect Control Hosp Epidemiol.* 2020:1-2.

22. Konda A, Prakash A, Moss GA, Schmoldt M, Grant GD, Guha S. Aerosol filtration efficiency of common fabrics used in respiratory cloth masks. *ACS Nano.* 2020;14(5):6339-6347.

23. Clase CM, Fu EL, Joseph M, et al. Cloth masks may prevent transmission of COVID-19: An evidence-based, risk-based approach. *Ann Intern Med.* 2020.

24. McLure HA, Mannam M, Talboys CA, Azadian BS, Yentis SM. The effect of facial hair and sex on the dispersal of bacteria below a masked subject. *Anaesthesia.* 2000;55(2):173-176.

25. Parker-Pope T. How Not to Wear a Mask. *The New York Times.* www.nytimes.com/2020/04/08/well/live/coronavirus-face-mask-mistakes.html. Published April 8, 2020. Accessed June 24, 2020.

26. Bothra A, Das S, Singh M, Pawar M, Maheswari A. Retroauricular dermatitis with vehement use of ear loop face masks during COVID-19 pandemic. *Journal of the European Academy of Dermatology and Venereology.* 2020.

27. Xie Z, Yang YX, Zhang H. Mask-induced contact dermatitis in handling COVID-19 outbreak. *Contact Dermatitis.* 2020.

28. Yan Y, Chen H, Chen L, et al. Consensus of Chinese experts on protection of skin and mucous membrane barrier for health-care workers fighting against coronavirus disease 2019. *Dermatol Ther.* 2020:e13310.

29. Bhatia R, Sindhuja T, Bhatia S, et al. Iatrogenic dermatitis in times of COVID-19: A pandemic within a pandemic. *J Eur Acad Dermatol Venereol.* 2020.

30. Chin AWH, Chu JTS, Perera MRA, et al. Stability of SARS-CoV-2 in different environmental conditions. *The Lancet Microbe.* 2020;1(1).

31. Ren SY, Wang WB, Hao YG, et al. Stability and infectivity of coronaviruses in inanimate environments. *World J Clin Cases.* 2020;8(8):1391-1399.

32. World Health Organization. Coronavirus disease (COVID-19) advice for the public. https://www.who.int/emergencies/diseases/novel-coronavirus-2019/advice-for-public. Updated June 4, 2020. Accessed July 20, 2020.

33. World Health Organization. Considerations for quarantine of individuals in the context of containment for coronavirus disease (COVID-19): interim guidance, 29 February 2020. World Health Organization;2020.

34. Centers for Disease Contol and Prevention. Cleaning and Disinfection for Households. https://www.cdc.gov/coronavirus/2019-ncov/prevent-getting-sick/cleaning-disinfection.html. Published 2020. Updated July 10, 2020. Accessed July 20, 2020.

35. Karamouzian M, Johnson C, Kerr T. Public health messaging and harm reduction in the time of COVID-19. *Lancet Psychiatry.* 2020;7(5):390-391.
36. Eslami H, Jalili M. The role of environmental factors to transmission of SARS-CoV-2 (COVID-19). *AMB Express.* 2020;10(1):92.
37. La Rosa G, Bonadonna L, Lucentini L, Kenmoe S, Suffredini E. Coronavirus in water environments: Occurrence, persistence and concentration methods - A scoping review. *Water Res.* 2020;179:115899.
38. Gu J, Han B, Wang J. COVID-19: gastrointestinal manifestations and potential fecal–oral transmission. *Gastroenterology.* 2020;158(6):1518-1519.

WHO IS AT RISK?

Which groups are considered high risk for infection with SARS-CoV-2?

People at high risk for infection with SARS-CoV-2 are older patients and those with a weakened immune system.[1-3] Regardless of age, patients with decreased immune function are at an increased risk of contracting COVID-19. Those who are immunosuppressed or immunodeficient are at a higher risk of catching COVID-19 as well. To find out if you are at risk of being immunocompromised and possibly at increased risk of catching COVID-19, speak with your doctor.

Which groups are considered high risk for severe COVID-19 outcomes?

People at high risk for severe disease (requiring hospitalization) are those suffering from chronic health problems, such as hypertension, diabetes, and obesity.[3-5] These health problems are frequently seen in patients with severe COVID-19 and may be an indicator for worse health outcomes.[4] COVID-19 can lead to an increased risk of death due to respiratory distress in these patient populations.[3,4] Older populations, those with chronic disease, and men are also more likely to experience severe health problems due to COVID-19 compared with younger patients, those without chronic disease, and women.[3,4,34-37]

Who is considered immunosuppressed?

Immunosuppression is when the immune system's ability to function is decreased, which leads to an increased risk of infection. Immunodeficiency or being immunocompromised are other ways of saying being immunosuppressed.

Some of the causes of immunosuppression include medication used to prevent rejection in transplant recipients or to treat autoimmune diseases, cancer treatment, and AIDS.[6-8] Immunosuppressed patients are at an increased risk for infection with viruses such as SARS-CoV-2 because of their body's dampened natural defense against foreign substances.[6,7] In the immunosuppressed patient population, it is important that patients follow CDC guidelines to help minimize their risk of contracting COVID-19.[8,9] Patients who are immunosuppressed should speak with their doctor about current treatments that may increase their chances of catching COVID-19. It is recommended that patients **not** stop their routine treatment because of COVID-19 unless advised to do so by their doctor.[9]

People can be immunodeficient because they are missing a component of their immune system.[10] Some patients with immunodeficiency may be more likely to be affected by viruses and may be at an increased risk of catching COVID-19.[10]

Which age groups are most likely to have a severe case?

It is more common for elderly patients (60 years or older) to experience severe health problems due to COVID-19.[1-4] This may be due to other underlying health problems these patients may have rather than being due to age alone. Older patients are more likely to suffer from hypertension, diabetes, and obesity (more information on controlled versus uncontrolled hypertension and diabetes in sections below) and are more likely to have a severe case of COVID-19 that requires hospitalization.[3-5] These health problems have also been associated with a higher mortality rate in patients hospitalized for COVID-19 compared with hospitalized patients without these health problems.[3,4]

Pediatric patients and young children are very likely to experience only mild symptoms from COVID-19.[5] However, it is possible for any age group to catch COVID-19, and there are cases of younger patients experiencing severe health problems related to COVID-19.[5] If a patient is experiencing symptoms of COVID-19 regardless of age, it is important they seek medical treatment to ensure the best health outcome.

Can infants catch COVID-19?

While young children are normally less susceptible to COVID-19 than adults, it is still possible for infants to catch COVID-19.[5,11-13] Infants exposed to an infected parent, caregiver, or contaminated environment may become infected.[11] The risk of infection of infants with SARS-CoV-2 can be decreased if those around infants follow safety protocols (e.g., wearing a mask, washing hands, no interaction with people with high exposure to SARS-CoV-2).[14] If you suspect your infant has been exposed to SARS-CoV-2 seek medical attention as soon as possible to mitigate any adverse health outcomes.

If an infant is exposed to SARS-CoV-2 and develops COVID-19, they should be checked by a medical professional to ensure they do not develop severe health effects. There have been several cases of COVID-19 associated with Kawasaki disease, and while there is currently little data to connect the two diseases, parents should be cautious.[15]Children with Kawasaki disease may experience fever, eye redness, swelling, rash, and swollen lymph nodes. Kawasaki disease may also cause heart disease in children because it causes dilation of blood vessels which may affect the coronary arteries.

Can kids catch COVID-19?

While it is less common for children to have a severe case of COVID-19, it is still possible for kids to become infected with SARS-CoV-2, often from an adult socially connected to the child (e.g., a parent or caregiver).[11] Kids may be asymptomatic carriers of SARS-CoV-2, meaning they have the virus and are contagious but show no symptoms of the disease. Children who are asymptomatic can spread the disease to other close contacts including adult relatives and other adult contacts.[11]

Does hypertension increase my risk?

There is a connection between hypertension and COVID-19 hospitalization.[2-4,16,17] A large percentage of patients hospitalized for COVID-19 also have hypertension.[2,3] SARS-CoV-2 viral particles may attach to a specific enzyme in the hypertensive pathway called angiotensin-converting enzyme (ACE), but further studies are needed to understand the importance of this pathway in the development of COVID-19.[16]

Patients with hypertension have worse outcomes when hospitalized with COVID-19.[2,3] Hypertension is one of a few health problems associated with COVID-19 death.[2,3] It is important for patients with hypertension to follow guidelines and take precautions to avoid exposure due to the increased risk of worse outcomes related to COVID-19.[2,3] If patients with hypertension develop symptoms of COVID-19, they should seek medical attention at their earliest convenience to ensure safety during the pandemic.

While following CDC guidelines is important for patients with hypertension to decrease their risk of COVID-19 infection, it is also important for patients to control their hypertension with prescribed medication. One study concluded patients taking ACE inhibitors or Angiotensin 2 receptor blockers (ARBs) for hypertension may have a lower risk of death due to COVID-19.[18] While more research is needed to validate if ACE inhibitors and ARBs decrease COVID-19 mortality in patients with hypertension, patients should follow their physician's guidance about taking medication for hypertension. Patients with hypertension should not stop taking their hypertension medication unless instructed to by their doctor.[18]

Does smoking increase my risk?

Currently, there are only limited data on the relationship between smoking and COVID-19.[19] While one research project stated smoking has the possibility to be helpful in protecting against COVID-19, far more research suggests smoking leads to worse outcomes in patients with COVID-19.[19-23] Some patients who smoke may have other health conditions (e.g., COPD) which make them more likely to suffer severe symptoms of

COVID-19.[22,23] More research is required to determine the effect of smoking on COVID-19.[19-23] However, smoking does lead to an increased risk of stroke and many forms of cancer.[24,25] Therefore, it is advised patients refrain from smoking to prevent other possible health problems.[24,25]

Does asthma increase my risk?

Asthma causes breathing difficulty, and respiratory viruses can cause asthma attacks to be worse than normal.[26,27] Currently, there are little data about asthma making patients more susceptible to infection with SARS-CoV-2.[26,28] Based on current data, patients with asthma are not at higher risk for developing COVID-19.[26, 27] However, patients with asthma who require a breathing tube (intubation) for COVID-19 tend to remain intubated for longer than patients without asthma.[29] More research is needed to assess whether asthma increases the risk of a patient becoming infected with SARS-CoV-2. Asthmatic patients can lower their exposure risk to SARS-CoV-2 by following their medication plan strictly to avoid asthma-related clinic or hospital visits .[26,27]

Does having an autoimmune disease increase my risk?

Autoimmunity is when the body's own immune system targets itself and causes damage. Currently, there is not enough research to determine whether patients with autoimmune diseases are at a higher risk of contracting COVID-19. However, how patients with autoimmune diseases are affected by other diseases may provide a clue. For example, patients with psoriasis suffer from pneumonia at a higher rate than patients without psoriasis.[30] Until more research is conducted, it is best for patients with an autoimmune disease to err on the side of caution and follow CDC guidelines and quarantine when possible. If you have an autoimmune disease and experience symptoms associated with COVID-19, you should seek medical treatment as soon as possible.

Lupus is an autoimmune disease in which the immune system attacks healthy cells and organs in the body, causing inflammation. A small study was performed to determine what effect lupus had on COVID-19 progression.[31] The lupus study was small, and no definitive trends could be concluded from it; however, based upon the limited data, the comorbidities associated with lupus may lead to more severe COVID-19.[31] While there is no current link between autoimmune conditions and increased risk of contracting COVID-19, patients should follow CDC guidelines.

COVID-19 may activate autoimmune conditions, specifically Guillain-Barré syndrome (GBS).[32] Viral diseases such as influenza, HIV, Zika, and SARS have triggered GBS.[32] GBS causes motor weakness, decreased sensation, and pain after a viral infection because it affects the nervous system.[32]

Does the treatment of autoimmune disease increase my risk?

Having an autoimmune disease being controlled by medication that dampens the body's natural immune system may, at least in theory, make a person more susceptible to COVID-19.[33] Medications for autoimmune diseases may suppress the immune system to stop the body's own immune system from hurting itself. The immune system is what helps protect against harmful organisms and viruses that enter the body; so when the immune system is not 100%, there is an increased risk of getting sick.[7] If people are taking medication for an autoimmune disease, they may be at an increased risk for catching COVID-19 and should follow CDC guidelines to lower their chances of getting COVID-19.[33]

Patients that are currently being treated for an autoimmune disease (e.g., psoriasis, rheumatoid arthritis, lupus) should not stop treatment due to fear of catching COVID-19.[34,35] Based on studies of patients on biologic therapies for psoriasis, biologic therapy may increase the risk of mild infection with SARS-CoV-2 but may also reduce the likelihood of severe COVID-19 and death.[35] In Italy, no deaths occurred in a study of almost 1,200 patients on biologic therapies for psoriasis.[35] Similar to dexamethasone—which is used to treat COVID-19—biologic therapies modulate the immune system and may reduce the likelihood of cytokine storm, which is a dangerous overactivation of the immune system.[34,35] Although there is still uncertainty and more research needs to be performed, immunosuppressive treatment may reduce the risk of serious outcomes.

Are men affected more often than women?

Men appear to be more susceptible to COVID-19 than women.[36-39] Older men above the age of 60 seem to have some of the worst outcomes when hospitalized for COVID-19, and this may be attributed to other health problems in this patient population.[36-39] Men who have hypertension and diabetes are at an increased risk for worse COVID-19 outcomes.[3-5] Why men are more likely to suffer from COVID-19 is still uncertain. One possibility is greater activity of the TMPRSS2 gene in males.[40] The TMPRSS2 gene regulates cellular machinery that helps in viral activation and entry into human cells which is needed by SARS-CoV, SARS-CoV-2, and influenza.[40]

Are minorities and people of color more likely to get COVID-19?

While COVID-19 has been devastating throughout the United States, minorities, including the African American population, may be more likely to get COVID-19.[41-43] While patient demographic data on COVID-19 cases have not been released for every state, there are some disturbing trends in the data which have been released.[41] In some states, the African American population—which makes up a minority of the total population—leads the state in number of confirmed COVID-19 cases.[41-43] The African American community in some states also has the most deaths due to COVID-19.[41-43]

A possible reason for this difference may be the increased prevalence of diabetes and obesity in African American communities due to environmental and socioeconomic factors.[44] In a study conducted in Bronx, New York, the African American population had an obesity rate of 36%, which may have contributed to the worse health outcomes of African Americans in the area during the COVID-19 pandemic.[44] However, the underlying reason for the high rate of obesity in the African American population in the study is unknown and may be attributed to environmental and socioeconomic factors.[44] Part of the study's patient population were economically challenged minorities, but the study did not discern if the patients were essential workers or not.[43]

Unfortunately, African Americans may not receive care for COVID-19 until their case has progressed to a more severe form leading to worse health outcomes.[45] Further research is needed to determine the factors that are causing minorities to disproportionately suffer from COVID-19, such as living and working conditions.

Does diabetes affect COVID-19 risk?

While research is still being conducted, it is believed that diabetes may lead to more severe COVID-19.[3,4] It is not yet known whether controlled diabetes or uncontrolled diabetes leads to worse COVID-19 outcomes. One study did assess the effects of diabetes and uncontrolled hyperglycemia (high blood sugar) in a study of patients hospitalized with COVID-19.[46] There was a higher rate of death from COVID-19 in the uncontrolled hyperglycemia group.[46] While this result is disturbing, the study did not consider other health problems the patients had besides their uncontrolled hyperglycemia.[46] Diabetics should be cautious, take their medication as pre-scribed, and try to maintain a normal blood sugar. Diabetic patients should follow CDC guidelines to avoid catching COVID-19. Patients with diabetes who have symptoms associ-ated with COVID-19 should seek medical attention as soon as possible because of their possible increased risk.

References

1. Liu K, Chen Y, Lin R, Han K. Clinical features of COVID-19 in elderly patients: A comparison with young and middle-aged patients. *J Infect.* 2020;80(6):e14–e18.
2. Du Y, Tu L, Zhu P, et al. Clinical features of 85 fatal cases of COVID-19 from Wuhan. A retrospective ob-

servational study. *Am J Respir Crit Care Med.*
2020;201(11):1372–1379.

3. Richardson S, Hirsch JS, Narasimhan M, et al. Presenting characteristics, comorbidities, and outcomes
among 5700 patients hospitalized with COVID-19 in
the New York City area [published online ahead of
print, 2020 Apr 22] [published correction appears in
doi: 10.1001/jama.2020.7681]. *JAMA.*
2020;323(20):2052–2059.

4. Zhou F, Yu T, Du R, et al. Clinical course and risk factors for mortality of adult inpatients with COVID-19
in Wuhan, China: a retrospective cohort study [pub-
lished correction appears in Lancet. 2020 Mar
28;395(10229):1038]. *Lancet.*
2020;395(10229):1054–1062.

5. Minotti C, Tirelli F, Barbieri E, Giaquinto C, Donà D.
How is immunosuppressive status affecting children
and adults in SARS-CoV-2 infection? A systematic review [published online ahead of print, 2020 Apr 23]. *J
Infect.* 2020;81(1): e61–e66.

6. Dropulic LK, Lederman HM. Overview of infections in
the immunocompromised host. *Microbiol Spectr.*
2016;4(4):10.1128/microbiolspec. DMIH2-0026-2016.

7. Zhu L, Xu X, Ma K, et al. Successful recovery of
COVID-19 pneumonia in a renal transplant recipient
with long-term immunosuppression [published online ahead of print, 2020 Mar 17]. *Am J Transplant.*
2020;10.1111/ajt.15869.

8. Al-Quteimat OM, Amer AM. The impact of the COVID-19 pandemic on cancer patients. *Am J Clin Oncol.* 2020;43(6):452–455.

9. Ceribelli A, Motta F, De Santis M, et al. Recommendations for coronavirus infection in rheumatic diseases treated with biologic therapy. *J Autoimmun.* 2020; 109:102442.

10. Raje N, Dinakar C. Overview of immunodeficiency disorders. *Immunol Allergy Clin North Am.* 2015;35(4):599-623.

11. Balasubramanian S, Rao NM, Goenka A, Roderick M, Ramanan AV. Coronavirus disease 2019 (COVID-19) in children - What we know so far and what we do not. *Indian Pediatr.* 2020;57(5):435–442.

12. Morand A, Fabre A, Minodier P, et al. COVID-19 virus and children: What do we know?. *Arch Pediatr.* 2020;27(3):117–118.

13. Hong H, Wang Y, Chung HT, Chen CJ. Clinical characteristics of novel coronavirus disease 2019 (COVID-19) in newborns, infants and children. *Pediatr Neonatol.* 2020;61(2):131–132.

14. Chen H, Guo J, Wang C, et al. Clinical characteristics and intrauterine vertical transmission potential of COVID-19 infection in nine pregnant women: a retrospective review of medical records [published correction appears in Lancet. 2020 Mar 28;395(10229):1038]. *Lancet.* 2020;395(10226):809–815.

15. Jones VG, Mills M, Suarez D, et al. COVID-19 and Kawasaki Disease: Novel virus and novel case. *Hosp Pediatr.* 2020;10(6):537–540.

16. Tadic M, Cuspidi C, Mancia G, Dell'Oro R, Grassi G. COVID-19, hypertension and cardiovascular diseases: Should we change the therapy? [published online ahead of print, 2020 May 13]. *Pharmacol Res.* 2020;158: 104906.

17. Zheng Z, Peng F, Xu B, et al. Risk factors of critical & mortal COVID-19 cases: A systematic literature review and meta-analysis [published online ahead of print, 2020 Apr 23]. *J Infect.* 2020; S0163-4453(20)30234-6.

18. Zhang P, Zhu L, Cai J, et al. Association of inpatient use of angiotensin-converting enzyme inhibitors and angiotensin II receptor blockers with mortality among patients with hypertension hospitalized with COVID-19. *Circ Res.* 2020;126(12):1671-1681.

19. Patanavanich R, Glantz SA. Smoking is associated with COVID-19 progression: A Meta-Analysis [published online ahead of print, 2020 May 13]. *Nicotine Tob Re*s. 2020; ntaa082.

20. Farsalinos K, Barbouni A, Niaura R. Systematic review of the prevalence of current smoking among hospitalized COVID-19 patients in China: could nicotine be a therapeutic option? [published online ahead of print, 2020 May 9]. *Intern Emerg Med.* 2020;1–8.

21. Lippi G, Henry BM. Active smoking is not associated with severity of coronavirus disease 2019 (COVID-19). *Eur J Intern Med.* 2020; 75:107–108.

22. Zhao Q, Meng M, Kumar R, et al. The impact of COPD and smoking history on the severity of COVID-19: A systemic review and meta-analysis [published online ahead of print, 2020 Apr 15]. J *Med Virol.* 2020;10.1002/jmv.25889.

23. Alqahtani JS, Oyelade T, Aldhahir AM, et al. Prevalence, severity and mortality associated with COPD and smoking in patients with COVID-19: A rapid systematic review and meta-analysis. *PLoS One.* 2020;15(5):e0233147. Published 2020 May 11.

24. Pan B, Jin X, Jun L, Qiu S, Zheng Q, Pan M. The relationship between smoking and stroke: A meta-analysis. *Medicine* (Baltimore). 2019;98(12):e14872.

25. de Groot P, Munden RF. Lung cancer epidemiology, risk factors, and prevention. *Radiol Clin North Am.* 2012;50(5):863–876.

26. Morais-Almeida M, Aguiar R, Martin B, et al. COVID-19, asthma, and biologic therapies: What we need to know [published online ahead of print, 2020 May 16]. *World Allergy Organ J.* 2020;13(5):100126.

27. Liu S, Zhi Y, Ying S. COVID-19 and Asthma: Reflection during the pandemic [published online ahead of print, 2020 May 28]. *Clin Rev Allergy Immunol.* 2020;10.1007/s12016-020-08797-3.

28. Pennington E. Asthma increases risk of severity of COVID-19 [published online ahead of print, 2020 May 5]. *Cleve Clin J Med.* 2020;10.3949/ccjm.87a.ccc002.

29. Mahdavinia M, Foster KJ, Jauregui E, et al. Asthma prolongs intubation in COVID-19 [published online

ahead of print, 2020 May 14]. *J Allergy Clin Immunol Pract.* 2020; S2213-2198(20)30476-1.

30. Kao LT, Lee CZ, Liu SP, Tsai MC, Lin HC. Psoriasis and the risk of pneumonia: a population-based study. *PLoS One.* 2014;9(12):e116077. Published 2014 Dec 26.

31. Mathian A, Mahevas M, Rohmer J, et al. Clinical course of coronavirus disease 2019 (COVID-19) in a series of 17 patients with systemic lupus erythematosus under long-term treatment with hydroxychloroquine. *Ann Rheum Dis.* 2020;79(6):837-839.

32. Dalakas MC. Guillain-Barré syndrome: The first documented COVID-19-triggered autoimmune neurologic disease: More to come with myositis in the offing. Neurol Neuroimmunol *Neuroinflamm.* 2020;7(5):e781. Published 2020 Jun 9.

33. Sarzi-Puttini P, Marotto D, Antivalle M, et al. How to handle patients with autoimmune rheumatic and inflammatory bowel diseases in the COVID-19 era: An expert opinion. *Autoimmun Rev.* 2020;19(7):102574.

34. Bashyam AM, Feldman SR. Should patients stop their biologic treatment during the COVID-19 pandemic. *J Dermatolog Treat.* 2020;31(4):317-318.

35. Damiani G, Pacifico A, Bragazzi NL, Malagoli P. Biologics increase the risk of SARS-CoV-2 infection and hospitalization, but not ICU admission and death: Real-life data from a large cohort during red-zone declaration [published online ahead of print, 2020 May 1]. *Dermatol Ther.* 2020; e13475.

36. Shi H, Han X, Jiang N, et al. Radiological findings from 81 patients with COVID-19 pneumonia in

Wuhan, China: a descriptive study. *Lancet Infect Dis.* 2020;20(4):425–434.

37. Yi Y, Lagniton PNP, Ye S, Li E, Xu RH. COVID-19: what has been learned and to be learned about the novel coronavirus disease. *Int J Biol Sci.* 2020;16(10):1753–1766. Published March 15, 2020.

38. Chen T, Wu D, Chen H, et al. Clinical characteristics of 113 deceased patients with coronavirus disease 2019: retrospective study [published correction appears in BMJ. 2020 Mar 31;368:m1295]. *BMJ.* 2020;368:m1091. Published 2020 Mar 26.

39. Cozzi D, Albanesi M, Cavigli E, et al. Chest X-ray in new coronavirus disease 2019 (COVID-19) infection: findings and correlation with clinical outcome [published online ahead of print, 2020 Jun 9]. *Radiol Med.* 2020;1–8.

40. Stopsack KH, Mucci LA, Antonarakis ES, Nelson PS, Kantoff PW. TMPRSS2 and COVID-19: Serendipity or opportunity for intervention?. *Cancer Discov.* 2020;10(6):779-782.

41. Brandt EB, Beck AF, Mersha TB. Air pollution, racial disparities, and COVID-19 mortality [published online ahead of print, 2020 May 7]. *J Allergy Clin Immunol.* 2020; S0091-6749(20)30632-1.

42. Fouad MN, Ruffin J, Vickers SM. COVID-19 is out of proportion in African Americans. This will come as no surprise... [published online ahead of print, 2020 May 19]. *Am J Med.* 2020;S0002-9343(20)30411-3.

43. Mahajan UV, Larkins-Pettigrew M. Racial demographics and COVID-19 confirmed cases and deaths: a cor-

relational analysis of 2886 US counties [published online ahead of print, 2020 May 21]. *J Public Health (Oxf)*. 2020; fdaa070.

44. Palaiodimos L, Kokkinidis DG, Li W, et al. Severe obesity, increasing age and male sex are independently associated with worse in-hospital outcomes, and higher in-hospital mortality, in a cohort of patients with COVID-19 in the Bronx, New York. *Metabolism*. 2020; 108:154262.

45. Azar KMJ, Shen Z, Romanelli RJ, et al. Disparities in outcomes among COVID-19 patients in a large health care system in California [published online ahead of print, 2020 May 21]. *Health Aff* (Millwood). 2020;101377hlthaff202000598.

46. Bode B, Garrett V, Messler J, et al. Glycemic characteristics and clinical outcomes of COVID-19 patients hospitalized in the United States [published correction appears in *J Diabetes Sci Technol*. 2020 Jun 10:1932296820932678]. J Diabetes Sci Technol. 2020;14(4):813-821.

AVOIDING MISINFORMATION

Where should I go for reliable information on the COVID-19 pandemic from a global perspective?

There is an abundance of false information regarding COVID-19 available on the internet, so make sure you are using reputable sources by checking out global, national, and local health services' websites. The World Health Organization (WHO) is one of the largest and most trusted public health entities, and since COVID-19 is a global pandemic, the WHO is following the virus and its international effects closely. The WHO website (www.who.int/emergencies/diseases/novel-coronavirus-2019) offers guidelines and general advice for the public.[1]

Where should I go for reliable information on COVID-19 in the United States?

Refer to the Centers for Disease Control and Prevention (CDC) website (www.cdc.gov/coronavirus) for nationwide updates regarding COVID-19. The CDC offers information regarding symptoms, testing, prevention, data and surveillance, guidance, and more.[2] The CDC also offers statistics on cases and deaths at the country, state, and county level.

The National Institutes of Health (NIH) is another reliable source of information. The NIH website (www.nih.gov/coronavirus) provides up-to-date national news on treatment guidelines, potential vaccines, and COVID-19 testing. This organization is a good resource for updates in research and scientific breakthroughs regarding the virus; for example, the NIH announced the halt in hydroxychloroquine clinical trials.[3]

The Food and Drug Administration (FDA) is an agency within the U.S. Department of Health and Human Services. It works to protect public health through the regulation of food, drugs, medical devices, and vaccines. Visit the FDA website (www.fda.gov) for updates on COVID-19 testing, personal protective equipment (PPE), drug and medical device advancements, and proactive advice regarding infection prevention and recovery from COVID-19. For example, in early July the FDA warned consumers about hand sanitizers contaminated with methanol, a toxic form of alcohol that can be absorbed through the skin. The FDA then posted a list of these methanol-containing products on its website.[4]

How can I stay up to date on COVID-19 recommendations in my hometown?

For local information regarding COVID-19 and its effects in your state, check the CDC's website for a directory of state and territorial health departments (www.cdc.gov/publichealthgateway/healthdirectories/healthdepartments.html). This directory lists websites for each state's Department of Public

Health, which provides local updates and information regarding COVID-19 precautions in your hometown.[5]

Each state's Department of Public Health can also be reached through the CDC's COVID Data Tracker (www.cdc.gov/covid-data-tracker), which is an interactive map that shows case statistics by state. Clicking an individual state will navigate to its local health department website.

What are statistical models?

Statistical models are a mathematical representation of data and information. They attempt to predict outcomes based on established information, generating assumptions based on a set of input variables. Simple models may have only a few variables, while more complex models may incorporate thousands of variables. Statistical models are being used in the COVID-19 pandemic to estimate and analyze the virus's impact on society, such as how many people will be infected and how unemployment rates will fluctuate.

Why do statistical models vary so much?

Statistical models incorporate varying information into their projections, so the outcome of each model depends on what information is put into it. A model may incorporate the infectivity of the virus and how it spreads and evolves, or it may focus on the immune system's response to the virus, whether immunity develops, and whether that immunity is effective. Differing rates of disease spread among urban and rural areas, varying healthcare systems, and public reactions to the pandemic may also be reflected in models. Models vary in reliability since they attempt to reflect an accurate picture of society, which becomes incredibly difficult with increasing numbers of variables.[6]

Furthermore, depending on the specific point in time that a model is made, projected outcomes will differ. For example, in March 2020, the Imperial College London model predicted that over 2.2 million deaths would occur in the United States if no action was taken to curb the spread of the virus. In response to this prediction, the United States imposed a lockdown and advised social distancing, which changed the predicted number of deaths. This inability to predict the public response to new data was a limitation that made the model less accurate.

In comparison, the statistical model put forth by the Institute for Health Metrics and Evaluation is frequently updated to adjust for changes in social distancing, testing variability, and data availability. This model takes into consideration the changing environment we live in to adjust projected deaths. However, this interplay between prediction and reaction is difficult to determine. In sum, statistical models vary widely because they can only reflect data that is put into them, a global pandemic is an extraordinarily complex situation, and public behaviors change—sometimes unpredictably.[6]

How can I tell if I am reading trustworthy information?

With the immense amount of information available regarding COVID-19, it is important to make sure that your information comes from a reliable source. Look for citations that detail where the information comes from. For research, look at where the research was published. Peer-reviewed journals such as *JAMA* and national organizations such as the CDC tend to be reliable sources. Major academic institutions are usually a reliable source of evidence-based updates regarding COVID-19.[7]

Avoid depending on social media for COVID-19 updates; anyone can post information that may go viral, and viral does not necessarily mean true. Notable exceptions include the WHO and CDC, which both have social media accounts that provide accurate information (the WHO provides links to all of its social media accounts at the bottom of its home page, www.who.int, and the CDC's social media accounts are listed at www.cdc.gov/socialmedia/index.html). Always double-check where information is from to avoid pseudoscience and disinformation.

What are some indicators of untrustworthy information?

There are several steps you can take to identify an untrustworthy source of information. First, look at the tone of the article. Untrustworthy sources often have an overtly political, volatile, or biased tone. Next, see if there are citations and valid references. If the information lacks a citation or has an illegitimate citation, it is less likely to be reliable. The legitimacy of citations can be checked by looking up the reference and ensuring that the article or resource actually exists. Then, look at the author's information. If the author uses a pseudonym or alias, they may not be sharing valid information. Trustworthy scientific information is rarely—if ever—published under cover of a pseudonym.[7] Finally, ask if the information is trying to sell a product or service. Marketing disguised as information is generally not reliable.

Correctly identifying information as trustworthy or not takes time and practice, but it is a worthwhile skill to learn and becomes easier over time.

I heard that the virus came from a market, a lab, then bats. What facts are known about the cause of this pandemic?

There are many false rumors surrounding the origin of SARS-CoV-2, the virus that causes COVID-19. However, it is established that in December 2019 China reported an outbreak of pneumonia of unknown cause to the WHO. By January 30, 2020, the WHO deemed the outbreak a Public Health Emergency of International Concern.[8]

Based on genetic analysis of SARS-CoV-2, the virus appears to have originated in bats. However, it is not yet clear how the virus was transmitted from bats to humans; another animal may have served as an "intermediate host" before the virus began to infect humans.[9] While SARS-CoV-2 may not have originally emerged in the Wuhan wet market—a market which sells fresh meat, produce, and where animals are slaughtered—the market clearly served as an epidemiological source by amplifying the virus and allowing it to take hold. Approximately two-thirds of the earliest cases in Wuhan, China, had contact with the market in question.[9] Although we do not know the precise origin of SARS-CoV-2 with certainty, there is no credible evidence supporting the theory that the virus was manufactured in a lab. This bioterrorism rumor started because of similarities between HIV and SARS-CoV-2, but it was disproven after analysis of the viral genomes concluded that the only similarities were due to random chance.[10]

I heard that heat kills coronaviruses. Can I use a hairdryer to disinfect things?

Hairdryers and hand dryers should not be used for disinfection. The best way to disinfect surfaces is by using soap and water, a detergent followed by sodium hypochlorite (chlorine bleach), or alcohol disinfectant. Bleach should not be used on skin and should never be injected or ingested.[11]

Heat at 56°C will kill the SARS coronavirus in a laboratory environment but changing environmental conditions can make the viral particles less susceptible to heat.[12] However, no comparable studies have been done to determine the amount of heat needed to kill SARS-CoV-2 outside of the lab. So, while a high-powered hairdryer or heat gun could potentially kill coronavirus on a surface, this method of disinfection has not been proven effective against SARS-CoV-2, and it is safer and more efficient to use soap and water or alcohol disinfectant.

Additionally, hairdryers vary in power and it is difficult to concentrate and measure the heat they emit. Hairdryers can cause significant burning when applied to skin, which may increase susceptibility to SARS-CoV-2 by damaging the body's natural defenses and barriers. Using a hair dryer on your nose or mouth will not prevent COVID-19 because once the virus has attached itself to a mucous membrane—such as that in the nose or mouth—the virus is already replicating and infecting.[13]

Will taking a hot bath or shower kill COVID-19?

If you have been infected by SARS-CoV-2, meaning the virus has entered your body, bathing in hot water will not prevent COVID-19 because your internal body temperature does not change when you sit in a hot bath or shower. However, the hot water can burn your skin, so this is not advised.[14]

If SARS-CoV-2 is on your skin or you have touched a contaminated surface, simply using alcohol-based hand sanitizer or handwashing with soap and water is the most effective way to remove the virus. This will decrease your chances of inadvertently infecting yourself.

Can COVID-19 be transmitted in areas with hot, humid climates?

Yes. Hot or cold climates do not kill SARS-CoV-2. Countries with hot climates are still reporting COVID-19 cases, and warmer weather is not predicted to slow the spread of the virus.[13] Based on data from nations in the tropics and Southern Hemisphere, which were initially affected in their summer season, hot weather has little effect on slowing the spread of the virus.[15] This is likely due to the remaining high susceptibility among people worldwide; early in the pandemic, nobody had immunity to the virus so everyone was susceptible.[15] This near-universal susceptibility allows SARS-CoV-2 to spread rapidly.

I heard that ultraviolet (UV) light kills coronaviruses. Can I use UV light to disinfect things?

Although UV light is an effective disinfectant when used properly and at the right wavelength, it should not be used on the skin or body since hand washing and hand sanitizers are more effective at removing the virus.[16] Some hospitals are using UV light to disinfect masks and gowns, but evidence supporting this practice is limited since it is difficult to measure the exact time and dosage needed to disinfect an object with grooves and wrinkles such as a hospital gown. Additionally, UV light can cause skin and eye damage. Using a home UV light is not advised since there are no data that suggest that this prevents COVID-19, and there are significant safety hazards associated with home UV light use.[16]

Are there any supplements that will prevent me from getting sick?

Currently, there are no medications or supplements proven to prevent or cure COVID-19. Despite rumors, there is no evidence that garlic, vitamin C, essential oils, or probiotics help prevent COVID-19.[17] The FDA is a reliable source of information that debunks myths—which often trend on social media—regarding supplements which prevent COVID-19 (www.fda.gov/consumers/health-fraud-scams/fraudulent-coronavirus-disease-2019-covid-19-products).

Some potentially helpful vitamins and minerals are under investigation. Zinc is a mineral that is vital to immune system function, and trials are underway to study its effects on preventing COVID-19. A few reports have associated increased rates of COVID-19 infection and death with low vitamin D levels, and data from China have shown a lower death rate from COVID-19 in areas of high selenium intake. However, association does not mean causation, and there is no reliable evidence that zinc, vitamin D, or selenium supplementation prevent infection or death from COVID-19. In summary, no supplement has demonstrated efficacy in preventing or curing COVID-19.[18]

I heard that I can get COVID-19 from letters and packages. Is this true?

The risk of getting COVID-19 from mail and other packages is low. An infected person's respiratory droplets would have to contaminate the package first, and the material the package is made from affects the viability of the virus.

In laboratory conditions, SARS-CoV-2 can survive on stainless steel and plastics longer than on cardboard and copper. On plastic, the half-life of viability is estimated to be 6.8 hours. This means that after 6.8 hours on plastic, the number of viral particles will have decreased by half.[19] The virus can remain viable for up to three days on plastic and stainless steel surfaces. In contrast, copper surfaces decrease the lifespan of SARS-CoV-2 to a maximum of four hours.[18]

Although it is unlikely to contract COVID-19 through packaging, it is not impossible. Being proactive by disposing of outer packaging promptly, waiting a few hours, or spraying plastic packaging with a disinfectant before handling—followed by washing your hands—are all effective ways of decreasing transmission through touching potentially contaminated surfaces such as mail.

Should I use a nasal rinse or wash?

No. There is no scientific data supporting the use of nasal rinses to prevent COVID-19. Limited evidence suggests that regularly rinsing with saline can protect people from the common cold, but that is the extent of its protection. There is no support of this prophylactic measure when it comes to respiratory infections such as COVID-19. This is likely since SARS-CoV-2 begins replicating and infecting immediately upon contact with the nasal mucosa.[13]

Do 5G mobile networks cause COVID-19?

Definitely not. Viruses cannot travel through radio waves or mobile networks. Additionally, COVID-19 has spread in developing countries and areas that lack 5G coverage. SARS-CoV-2 spreads through the inhalation of respiratory droplets, which are produced when an infected person sneezes, coughs, or speaks. These droplets can also land on surfaces, contaminating them, and then cause infection when another person touches the surface before touching their mouth, nose, or eyes.[13] Mobile networks have no role in the spread of infectious diseases.

References

1. World Health Organization. Coronavirus disease (COVID-19) advice for the public. https://www.who.int/emergencies/diseases/novel-coronavirus-2019/advice-for-public. Updated April 29, 2020. Accessed June 6, 2020.

2. Centers for Disease Control and Prevention. Coronavirus (Covid-19). https://www.cdc.gov/coronavirus/2019-nCoV/index.html. Updated June 05, 2020. Accessed June 6, 2020.

3. National Institutes of Health. Coronavirus (Covid-19). https://www.nih.gov/health- information/coronavirus. Reviewed May 14, 2020. Accessed June 6, 2020.

4. U.S. Food and Drug Administration. Coronavirus disease 2019 (COVID-19). https://www.fda.gov/emergency-preparedness-and-response/counterterrorism-and-emerging- threats/coronavirus-

disease-2019-covid-19#ppe. Updated June 05, 2020. Accessed June 6, 2020.

5. Centers for Disease Control and Prevention. Public Health Professionals Gateway. https://www.cdc.gov/publichealthgateway/healthdirectories/healthdepartments.html. Updated May 01, 2020. Accessed June 6, 2020.

6. Holmdahl I, Buckee C. Wrong but useful -- What Covid-19 epidemiologic models can and cannot tell us. *New England Journal of Medicine*. May 2020.

7. Katellak K. A COVID-19 'Infodemic'? How to make sense of what you're reading. Yale Medicine. https://www.yalemedicine.org/stories/covid-19-infodemic. Published April 13, 2020. Accessed June 6, 2020.

8. World Health Organization. Rolling updates on coronavirus disease (Covid-19). https://www.who.int/emergencies/diseases/novel-coronavirus-2019/events-as-they-happen. Updated June 01, 2020. Accessed June 6, 2020.

9. Mackenzie JS, Smith DW. COVID-19: a novel zoonotic disease caused by a coronavirus from China: what we know and what we don't. *Microbiol Aust*. 2020; MA20013.

10. Liu SL, Saif LJ, Weiss SR, Su L. No credible evidence supporting claims of the laboratory engineering of SARS-CoV-2. *Emerg Microbes Infect*. 2020;9(1):505-507.

11. World Health Organization. Q&A: Considerations for the cleaning and disinfection of environmental sur-

faces in the context of COVID-19 in non-health care settings. https://www.who.int/emergencies/diseases/novel-coronavirus-2019/question-and-answers-hub/q-a- detail/q-a-considerations-for-the-cleaning-and-disinfection-of-environmental-surfaces-in-the-context- of-covid-19-in-non-health-care-settings. Published May 16, 2020. Accessed June 6, 2020.

12. Rabenau HF, Cinatl J, Morgenstern B, Bauer G, Preiser W, Doerr HW. Stability and inactivation of SARS coronavirus. *Med Microbiol Immunol.* 2005;194(1-2):1-6.

13. World Health Organization. Coronavirus disease (COVID-19) advice for the public: Myth busters. https://www.who.int/emergencies/diseases/novel-coronavirus-2019/advice-for-public/myth-busters. Published April 27, 2020. Accessed June 6, 2020.

14. Harvard T.H. Chan School of Public Health. Myths vs facts. https://www.hsph.harvard.edu/india- center/myths-vs-facts. Accessed June 6, 2020.

15. Kelly M. Local climate unlikely to drive the early COVID-19 pandemic. Princeton University. https://www.princeton.edu/news/2020/05/18/local-climate-unlikely-drive-early-covid-19-pandemic. Published May 18, 2020. Accessed June 6, 2020.

16. MedicineNet News. Can UV light kill or prevent coronavirus? https://www.medicinenet.com/can_uv_light_kill_or_prevent_coronavirus-news.htm. Published May 21, 2020. Accessed June 6, 2020.

17. Fortin J. That 'Miracle Cure' you saw on Facebook? It won't stop the coronavirus. The New York Times website. https://www.nytimes.com/2020/03/18/

health/coronavirus-cure-gargle-water.html. Published
March 18, 2020. Accessed June 6, 2020.

18. Cleveland Clinic. Supplements won't prevent or treat
Covid-19. https://health.clevelandclinic.org/no- sup-
plements-wont-prevent-or-treat-covid-19. Published
June 05, 2020. Accessed June 6, 2020.

19. van Doremalen N, Bushmaker T, Morris DH, et al.
Aerosol and surface stability of SARS-CoV-2 as compared with SARS-CoV-1. *New England Journal of Medicine.* 2020; 382:1564-1567.

WORK, SCHOOL, AND THE OFFICE

I work in an office with other people. What precautions can I take, as an employee or employer?

If working from home is not possible, or your workplace has started to reopen, there are several precautions that you can take in addition to standard social distancing guidelines. Many precautions are available, and your ability to implement them will depend on your specific workplace—taking some precautions is better than taking none. Although it is not clear how often COVID-19 is transmitted through contaminated surfaces, it is better to be safe than sorry.[1] The following methods can be used to reduce risk in the workplace, and following even a few will help to reduce the risk of workplace transmission.

- **Common areas:**
  -Require face masks to be worn properly at all times

while in buildings[2]

-Check temperatures of everyone at entrances

-Set maximum capacities for conference rooms, break rooms, and other communal areas

-Discourage in-person meetings by removing chairs from conference rooms

-Encourage virtual and phone meetings

-Reduce the number of people on site by having employees come in on rotating weekdays (e.g., some come only on Mondays, some only on Tuesdays, etc.)

-Increase the number of hand sanitizer stations (if possible, have contactless automatic dispensers or activation via foot pedal)

-Limit hallway conversations to five minutes or less

-Encourage people to take the stairs, instead of elevators, when possible

-Maintain social distancing in common areas like elevators, staircases, escalators, and hallways

· **Cubicles:**

-Convert every other cubicle to storage space to promote social distancing

-Remove equipment, chairs, and phones from storage cubicles to discourage people from sitting at them

-Outfit remaining cubicles with universal laptop docks, keyboards, mice, and monitors to create completely depersonalized "hotel" cubes

-Employees are responsible for wiping down each workspace before and after using a hotel cube

-Implement a booking system that requires employees to book a cube prior to using it—this will allow for contact tracing

-Have cubicles deep cleaned and disinfected daily

- **Cafeteria:**
  -Offer pre-packaged lunches instead of open buffets
  -Implement an online ordering system to prevent queues
  -Implement cash-free exchanges or other contactless payment systems
  -Use stickers or tape on the ground to indicate a safe 6-foot distance and traffic flow
  -Tape off seats or tables to encourage distancing, or remove tables entirely
  -Separate different teams (e.g., engineers cannot enter the cafeteria at the same time as manufacturing) to prevent commingling
  -Stagger break times
  -Place hand sanitizing stations near vending machines, coffee machines, microwaves, and any other communal items

- **Bathrooms:**
  -Install automatic or foot-pedal toilets and faucets to reduce touch points
  -Tape off every other sink and urinal

- **Other:**
  -Encourage employees to work from home by implementing work-from-home (WFH)-friendly policies

-Provide data stipends for work-related data usage
-Institute leave policies that encourage workers to stay home when sick
-Offer reimbursement for work-from-home gear

Which jobs, outside of healthcare, have the most exposure to SARS-CoV-2?

Healthcare workers in any capacity are among the highest risk due to the nature of their jobs; however, any job that requires contact with other people will have some risk. Risk of exposure to SARS-CoV-2 is based on three attributes: how much contact is required to perform the job, physical proximity to others, and exposure to disease and infection.[3]

Among essential workers, teachers, correctional officers, firefighters, police officers, transportation workers, veterinarians, and flight attendants are all at high risk.[3] These jobs all require extensive interaction with the public and frequent verbal communication. In general, talking loudly or more frequently produces more respiratory droplets than talking quietly or not talking at all. Working in a school, prison, or as a flight attendant also requires spending extended periods of time with many people in a confined space.[3]

Among those considered non-essential workers, hairdressers, barbers, food preparation, and food service workers are at high risk.[3] Any job that requires frequent in-person communication or close physical proximity with other people will likely have high exposure to SARS-CoV-2.

Is it safe to have communal food? What about a shared fridge?

Although many bacteria can multiply in food, viruses—including SARS-CoV-2—are unable to do so.

Additionally, there are no known cases of COVID-19 transmission through food or food packaging.[4] While transmission is not known to occur through food, having communal food or a shared fridge increases the likelihood of people coming into contact with one another and increases the number of touch points in a shared space. Therefore, it is not recommended to offer communal food or buffet-style meals. Regardless, good hygiene practices—including handwashing and disinfecting frequently touched surfaces—should be followed to reduce the potential for transmission through contaminated objects.

What is the difference between cleaning and disinfecting?

Cleaning refers to the physical removal of dirt and germs from surfaces and can be done with soap and water. Disinfecting refers to killing germs and can be done with chemicals, high temperatures, or ultraviolet light. Cleaning should be done before disinfection since cleaning will remove visible dirt and make disinfection more effective. Properly cleaning and disinfecting greatly reduces the likelihood of spreading infectious diseases through the environment.

How frequently should offices and facilities be cleaned and/or disinfected?

More frequently used objects and surfaces, or those in public areas, will need to be cleaned more often than those that are private or rarely used. At a minimum, offices should be cleaned at least daily. Depending on volume of people and use of surfaces, the frequency of cleaning varies. For example, a public bathroom should be cleaned much more often than desks in an office since more people will use the public bathroom, more surfaces will be touched in the bathroom, and bathrooms are inherently dirtier than offices.

Disinfection should focus on high touch surfaces, such as doorknobs, handles, light switches, phones, keyboards, computer mice, faucets, cash registers, and checkout counters. Use common Environmental Protection Agency (EPA)-registered household disinfectants while cleaning these to reduce the risk of transmitting viruses and bacteria.

Is it safe to vacuum?

There are no documented cases of COVID-19 transmission through vacuuming.[7] However, vacuuming can re-suspend settled dust, exposing people to dust and other allergens.[8] Spread of infectious disease has occurred via vacuuming: in the 1950s, an outbreak of Salmonella in a children's hospital was attributed to a vacuum.[8] In addition, bacteria and mold have been recovered from vacuum dust bags, and vacuum emissions can release appreciable quantities of bacteria.[8] However, the spread of infectious disease through vacuuming is not a hot area of research. Therefore, it is best to be cautious when vacuuming areas that may be contaminated.

Vacuums should be equipped with high-efficiency particulate air (HEPA) filters, especially for the exhaust.[9] These filters should be cleaned or replaced regularly. Poorly sealed vacuums may spread SARS-CoV-2 if used in contaminated areas before clean areas. If you are vacuuming in a school, office, or community building, do not vacuum a room that has people in it, and consider turning off room fans to prevent the dispersion of any particles generated from vacuuming.[9] If you must clean a room where people with SARS-CoV-2 have been, consider waiting 24 hours before vacuuming.

Should offices have sneeze guards? Is the cubicle still an acceptable arrangement?

The cubicle is an acceptable arrangement if social distancing guidelines can still be upheld and employees wear masks. Data on whether sneeze guards (clear plastic or glass barriers) are effective at preventing the spread of SARS-CoV-2 are not available. The physical presence of a barrier may be helpful as a reminder to maintain a safe distance; however, the barrier may also offer a sense of false security, since this type of barrier does not offer any peripheral seal and permits air to flow freely around it. Regardless of whether a sneeze guard is used, people should be wearing masks. Universal and constant mask-wearing is almost certainly more effective at preventing disease than sneeze guards, since effective masks will catch the wearer's respiratory droplets before they are able to disperse.

Should offices and schools use special HEPA filters in their HVAC systems?

HVAC (heating, ventilation, and air conditioning) systems are responsible for indoor heating, cooling, humidity, filtration, and air exchange. In hospitals—particularly in intensive care units and operating rooms—these systems play a vital role in infection control by reducing the spread of airborne pathogens.[10] These environments use high efficiency particulate air (HEPA) filters to remove dust, pathogens, and other particles suspended in the air.[10]

There is little evidence that supports the use of these special filters in offices and schools, although they could potentially reduce transmission of disease.[11] Even the most effective air filtration systems will not prevent the spread of SARS-CoV-2 if an infected person is in the building, however, because people breathe more frequently than an HVAC system can filter the volume of air in a room. Regardless of whether HEPA filters are used in the HVAC system, a good HVAC system does not obviate the need for physical distancing, mask-wearing, handwashing, and other hygiene practices. These are always the first defense against infection.

When will it be safe to open schools and universities?

Ultimately, schools and universities will not return to a normal level of risk until herd immunity is achieved either through vaccination or natural infection. Herd immunity is when enough people in a population have immunity to a disease to limit the disease's spread; for more details on the concept of herd immunity, refer to Chapter 10, "Vaccines." However, if community transmission is low in an area and a robust contact tracing system is in place, it may be relatively safe to reopen schools with precautions in place.

Schools will require numerous infection control procedures that will likely require substantial increases in staff and funding. Students' and staff's temperatures will need to be checked upon entering buildings, janitorial staff will need to increase the frequency of cleaning and disinfection, more buses and bus drivers may be required to prevent crowding on buses, and class size may need to be reduced to allow students to keep their distance.[12] More teachers may be needed to accommodate these smaller class sizes.

In addition to these demands, it is particularly difficult to enforce social distancing among younger children. Although young children are unlikely to experience severe disease, they can be asymptomatic carriers and pose a risk to teachers, school staff, and parents.

Like the workplace, steps can be taken to reduce the risk associated with students physically returning to school[12]:

- Require students to wear masks
- Check the temperatures of everyone entering the building
- Rearrange classroom chairs
- Have students remain in one classroom throughout the day, instead of switching classrooms for each subject
- Have students eat lunch in classrooms instead of the cafeteria
- Implement online food ordering for students that buy lunch at school
- Tape markers on the floor 6 feet apart to encourage social distancing
- Hold classes in shifts (part in-person, part online) to reduce the number of students present at one time
- Clean and update HVAC systems

Are work-from-home (WFH) and virtual schooling here to stay?

Until an effective vaccine is developed and widely available, WFH and virtual schooling are probably here to stay. Ample technology exists that allows companies and schools to communicate virtually with students and employees. This greatly reduces social contacts and therefore the spread of COVID-19.

It is likely that WFH will become a permanent fixture for businesses that do not require an on-site presence. If productivity from WFH is comparable to working in-office, it is likely that the business environment will transform, as many companies will not want to pay rent or overhead costs associated with office buildings. Additionally, developments in on-line video conferencing and screen-sharing software are likely to contribute to an environment that is increasingly WFH-friendly.

Schools have a much tougher path. Virtual school is likely to become standard for the duration of the COVID-19 pandemic but will probably not become a new norm—particularly for younger students in primary school. Virtual schooling does not allow students to talk in-person with their teacher or socialize with friends throughout the day. Virtual school also eliminates opportunities to play on school sports teams, participate in clubs, play in music concerts, and go on field trips. In addition, younger children lose focus easily and get distracted from studies when their teacher is not physically in front of them. It is unreasonable to expect a kindergartner to remain focused on activities without direct supervision.

From a parent's perspective, virtual schooling may be problematic since parents have varying abilities to help their children with material and are often busy with work. Parents who must take time off from work to help their children with school may withdraw from the workforce and risk becoming financially insecure. In addition, students from families that cannot afford computers, textbooks, private tutoring, or other study materials will be at a greater disadvantage than students from families that can. Considering all these factors, virtual schooling is here for now, but it is probably not here to stay.

References

1. Centers for Disease Control and Prevention. Cleaning and Disinfection for Households. https://www.cdc.gov/coronavirus/2019-ncov/prepare/cleaning-disinfection.html. Published May 27, 2020. Accessed June 7, 2020.

2. Can face masks protect against the coronavirus? *Mayo Clinic.* https://www.mayoclinic.org/diseases-conditions/coronavirus/in-depth/coronavirus-mask/art-20485449. Published May 28, 2020. Accessed June 7, 2020.

3. Lu M. These are the occupations with the highest COVID-19 risk. World Economic Forum. https://www.weforum.org/agenda/2020/04/occupa-tions-highest-covid19-risk/. Published April 20, 2020. Accessed June 8, 2020.

4. Gurchiek K. Coronavirus: Taking precautions with food at work. *SHRM.* https://www.shrm.org/resource-sandtools/hr-topics/employee-relations/pages/coron-avirus-taking-precautions-with-food-at-work.aspx. Published March 18, 2020. Accessed June 9, 2020.

5. Will the coronavirus survive in the refrigerator or freezer?: FAQ. New Jersey COVID-19 Information Hub. https://covid19.nj.gov/faqs/coronavirus-information/about-novel-coronavirus-2019/will-the-coronavirus-

survive-in-the-refrigerator-or-freezer-u21gz2n7br. Published March 19, 2020. Accessed June 9, 2020.

6. Centers for Disease Control and Prevention. Cleaning and Disinfecting Your Facility. https://www.cdc.gov/coronavirus/2019-ncov/community/disinfecting-building-facility.html. Published April 14, 2020. Accessed June 10, 2020.

7. Centers for Disease Control and Prevention. Coronavirus (COVID-19) frequently asked questions. https://www.cdc.gov/coronavirus/2019-ncov/faq.html#Cleaning-and-Disinfection. Published June 2, 2020. Accessed June 10, 2020.

8. Veillette M, Knibbs LD, Pelletier A, et al. Microbial contents of vacuum cleaner bag dust and emitted bioaerosols and their implications for human exposure indoors. *Appl Environ Microbiol.* 2013;79(20):6331-6336. doi:10.1128/AEM.01583-13

9. Centers for Disease Control and Prevention. Environmental Services. https://www.cdc.gov/infectioncontrol/guidelines/environmental/background/services.html. Published May 14, 2019. Accessed July 10, 2020.

10. Saran S, Gurjar M, Baronia A, et al. Heating, ventilation and air conditioning (HVAC) in intensive care unit. *Crit Care.* 2020;24(1):194. Published May 6, 2020.

11. Dietz L, Horve PF, Coil DA, Fretz M, Eisen JA, Van Den Wymelenberg K. 2019 novel coronavirus (COVID-19) pandemic: Built environment considerations to reduce transmission [published correction appears in

mSystems. 2020 May 5;5(3):]. *mSystems.* 2020;5(2):e00245-20. Published April 7, 2020.

12. Centers for Disease Control and Prevention. Considerations for Schools. https://www.cdc.gov/coronavirus/2019-ncov/community/schools-childcare/schools.html. Published May 19, 2020. Accessed June 8, 2020.

TRAVEL: ESSENTIAL AND NON-ESSENTIAL

Is it safe to travel domestically?

Travel increases the risk of contracting and spreading COVID-19 and is therefore not advised unless absolutely necessary. The Centers for Disease Control and Prevention (CDC) encourages staying home because it is the best way to protect against the spread of COVID-19.[1] Although early cases in the United States were associated with travel to a high-risk country or close contact with a previously identified case, domestic travel is now one of the main drivers in community spread of COVID-19.[2] If you must travel, you can assess your risk by considering several factors of both your local and destination communities.

Investigate whether COVID-19 is spreading within the area you are planning to visit and if it is spreading within your local community. This can be accomplished using the CDC COVID Data Tracker website (www.cdc.gov/covid-data-tracker/#cases), which features a color-coded map of hot spot states and shows the number of new cases statewide over the past seven days. Clicking on a state will navigate to its local health department website, which offers even more detailed data. A case positivity rate of greater than 10% or more than 10 new cases per 100,000 residents over a seven-day rolling average suggests significant spread of COVID-19 in the area.[3] A seven-day rolling average is simply an average calculated from data from the last seven days; an average is used to capture the overall trend in case numbers because case numbers can fluctuate substantially day to day.

Your local community or destination may require a 14-day self-quarantine period after traveling, especially if you are traveling from an area with substantial community spread. This information can be obtained from state or local health department websites. Additionally, consider whether your travel arrangements will allow you to maintain a distance of 6 feet between yourself and others, as close contact increases the chance of human-to-human transmission of COVID-19.[4]

If I have to fly, where should I sit?

If you have to fly, the best seat is one that allows you to practice social distancing—in other words, try to keep a 6-foot distance between yourself and others, even on airplanes. While ideal, this may not be possible as airlines return to high volume domestic and international travel, and some airlines have resumed booking flights at full capacity.

It may be helpful to consider studies from past pandemics when picking a seat or trying to change seats. When examining the transmission of Severe Acute Respiratory Syndrome (SARS), another respiratory illness caused by a coronavirus, public health officials defined the zone of primary transmission as being within two rows of the infected person.[5] Primary transmission refers to contracting an illness directly from an infected person. This zone of primary transmission includes the row with the infected person, two rows in front of them, and two rows behind them. Passengers beyond this zone are still at risk of getting infected, but the risk is lower: passengers in the primary zone of transmission have approximately a 6% risk of getting infected, while those beyond this zone have approximately a 2% risk.

Other studies have examined the flight movement patterns of passengers and crew. Passengers in window seats are less likely to get up during a flight and thus less likely to be in close contact with those not in their row,[6] which decreases their chances of coming in contact with someone who is ill. Window seat passengers are also less exposed to aisle traffic relative to passengers seated more centrally.

Outside of seating choices, airlines are taking precautions to protect travelers. Airlines are working with the CDC and World Health Organization (WHO) to reduce customers' risk of catching COVID-19 no matter where they sit. These precautions include expanding cleaning procedures, requiring passengers to wear face masks, and adjusting inflight snack services.

If I have to fly, what precautions can I take?

Practicing hand and respiratory hygiene while traveling requires some advance preparation. Before leaving, pack sanitizing wipes and hand sanitizer that is least 60% alcohol and keep both within easy reach.[7] The TSA has made a special allowance to its liquid rules and is permitting passengers to bring one 12-ounce bottle of liquid hand sanitizer in their carry-on luggage.[8] Wash your hands with soap and water or hand sanitizer before leaving for the airport and again once you arrive. Other than that, the usual rules of social distancing apply: wear a face mask or cloth face covering at all times, avoid touching your face, and maintain a distance of 6 feet apart from others whenever possible.

Once you have boarded the aircraft, you can use antiseptic wipes to clean hard surfaces such as tray tables and armrests.[9] Opening the overhead air vents may be effective at preventing the spread of pathogens by catching infectious respiratory droplets in a downdraft that carries them to the floor.[10]

Generally, aircraft cabin air quality is quite good due to continuous filtration through high-efficiency particulate air (HEPA) filters, which capture greater than 99% of airborne microbes. These filters are similar to those used in hospital operating rooms and prevent bacteria, fungi, and viruses from lingering in the air. Recirculated, filtered air is combined with air from outside the aircraft, which at cruising altitudes is free of microorganisms.[11,12] Modern cabin air systems supply enough airflow to completely replace the cabin air volume 20 to 30 times per hour (20 to 30 air changes per hour).[13] Despite this constant filtration of air, it is still good practice to wear a mask and keep your distance from other passengers.

How risky are public transportation and ride-sharing services?

The risk associated with public transportation is currently unknown, given that no large studies have been performed. It is also difficult to trace cases to such a transient activity. However, there is some reassuring information from France: since cautiously reopening in May, over 150 clusters of

COVID-19—defined as three cases linked by contact—have been traced, and none have been linked to public transit.[14] Japan, which pursued aggressive contact tracing rather than strict lockdowns, had similar findings.[15] While this is promising, it is important to continue practicing respiratory and hand hygiene. Using public transportation is clearly not risk-free, but public transit may be lower risk than originally expected due to relatively short transit times, lack of conversation, and adherence to public health guidelines.

Ride-sharing services are an alternative to public transportation, although the risk of these services is similarly unknown. When using ride-share or taxi services, avoid contact with surfaces frequently touched by other passengers or the driver.[15] If offered free water, magazines, or other amenities, it may be best to politely decline them. Additionally, you can ask the driver to open the windows or turn the air conditioner to non-recirculation mode.[15]

How effective are temperature screens?

Temperature screens are not reliable at detecting people who are infected with SARS-CoV-2. These screens were implemented during prior public health emergencies to limit the spread of infection, and some places are again using temperature screens to prevent the spread of COVID-19.

While temperature screens are helpful in identifying people who are symptomatic, they do not catch asymptomatic carriers of the virus.[16] People who will bypass detection include those who are in the incubation period, those who have COVID-19 but do not develop a fever, and those who have taken antipyretic medications.[16] Temperature screens can provide a false sense of security because SARS-CoV-2 is transmissible even in the absence of symptoms. These screens are much more useful for illnesses such as Ebola which are transmissible only when a person is symptomatic.[17] Despite their limited utility, temperature screens are still widely used in businesses and public spaces.

If I have a fever, will I be allowed to fly?

Passengers with a fever, defined as a body temperature of 100.4° F (38° C) or greater, will most likely not be allowed to board aircraft. Some airlines are utilizing preflight checklists that require customers to self-assess for signs and symptoms of COVID-19, including fever, and if a customer has any symptoms the airline will ask that they reschedule their trip. Additionally, the CDC recommends that passengers with a fever—regardless of cause—avoid flying.[18]

The WHO has established guidelines for steps that should be taken if a traveler has a fever. Travelers should first be taken for an interview to determine the likelihood that the fever is due to exposure to SARS-CoV-2.[19] The interview will assess for signs and symptoms of COVID-19, and travelers will complete a Public Health Declaration form to obtain travel and contact history. If the signs and symptoms are indicative of COVID-19, the traveler should be isolated and then transferred to a healthcare facility. However, these are only guidelines, and in reality, the process may not follow this exact sequence.

When will it be safe to travel abroad?

Ultimately, international travel will not resume a normal level of risk until herd immunity is achieved. Many countries have put travel restrictions in place, closed borders, or enacted policies that reflect the risk of COVID-19 transmission from

international travel. For example, in March the U.S. Department of State posted a level 4 Global Health Advisory, which
advised U.S. citizens to avoid all international travel due to the
global impact of COVID-19.[20] Shortly after, the U.S. also began
restricting entry to the United States. These restrictions applied to foreign nationals from China, Iran, and all European
Union (E.U.) countries.[21]

In some cases, countries—or entire blocs of countries—have restricted travel from locations where the spread
of COVID-19 is poorly controlled. The E.U. opened its internal
borders in June, and in July the bloc began allowing visitors
from 15 other countries deemed safe, including South Korea,
New Zealand, and Rwanda. As of August 2020, the E.U. remains closed to visitors from the U.S., Russia, and Brazil,
where COVID-19 continues to spread rampantly.[9] The U.S. Department of State maintains an updated list of travel restrictions by country (www.travel.state.gov/content/travel/en/
traveladvisories/COVID-19-Country-Specific-Informa-
tion.html).

The absence of travel restrictions to a country does not im-
ply that traveling to said country is safe or advisable. Countries
whose economies rely heavily on tourism, in particular, may
not be able to sustain prolonged border closures. Caribbean
countries like Aruba began reopening in early July by allowing
entry of Canadian and European citizens.[22] Visitors must provide a negative SARS-CoV-2 test result within 72 hours of
arrival. For the foreseeable future, countries will have to mon-
itor and continuously reevaluate the spread of COVID-19 both
in-country and abroad when deciding how to proceed with
tourism.

What should I do if I get sick while abroad, and how can I prepare before traveling?

If you get sick while abroad, contact the nearest U.S. Embassy or Consulate.[23] Either can help navigate finding a healthcare facility or returning home. However, there are a few steps you can take prior to leaving the U.S. to be better prepared in the unfortunate circumstance you fall ill while abroad.

You can enroll in the Smart Traveler Enrollment Program (STEP), a free service that allows U.S. citizens and nationals to register their trip with the nearest U.S. Embassy or Consulate. Utilizing this program will provide you with safety updates regarding your destination country and is helpful in the event the U.S. embassy or your family needs to contact you during an emergency.[24]

Checking if your health insurance plan offers any international coverage is strongly advised. Some insurance companies will cover limited international care during emergencies but will provide more extensive coverage through add-on travel insurance plans. Medicare, on the other hand, usually does not cover health care received outside the U.S., U.S. territories, and U.S. territorial waters.[25] There are many nuances to insurance coverage, so it is best to contact your insurance company and see what your policy entails before deciding if you need to purchase short- or long-term travel insurance.

Is a safe vacation possible?

A safe vacation is still possible, and safety will depend on several factors: your mode of travel, your destination, and the activities you plan on doing.

First, how you travel can affect your risk. For example, traveling by airplane involves more exposure than traveling in a personal vehicle with family. Airports and airplanes have limited opportunities for social distancing from potentially infectious passengers, which is much less of an issue when traveling by car. However, traveling by car limits possible destinations, and exposure is still possible when stopping for gas, food, bathroom breaks, or at hotels.

Next, some destinations are riskier than others. In March and April of 2020, New York experienced exponential growth in COVID-19 cases, and then in June cases surged in Texas and Arizona as states began reopening. As states continue to lift restrictions, we will most likely see shifting hot spots which will affect where and when people want to travel. The CDC's COVID Data Tracker (www.cdc.gov/covid-data-tracker) offers up-to-date information on COVID cases within the U.S., and the WHO publishes daily situation reports (www.who.int/emergencies/diseases/novel-coronavirus-2019/situation-reports) that track cases by country.

Finally, the itinerary of your trip matters. Activities that involve close or long interactions with others are high risk for spreading SARS-CoV-2. Spending time indoors with other people—for example, dining in restaurants, drinking in bars, or visiting casinos—is much riskier than outdoor activities like hiking or camping. A low-risk vacation will take into account all three of these factors and might look like an outdoor adventure arrived at by car or a remote stay in an isolated area.

Is it safe to go on a cruise?

Cruises should be avoided while SARS-CoV-2 continues to spread. The CDC recommends deferring all cruise travel worldwide, especially among older adults and people with under-lying medical conditions, because cruises increase the risk of person-to-person transmission of infectious diseases includ-ing COVID-19.[26] On the Diamond Princess cruise ship, during one of the earliest outbreaks of the pandemic, the basic repro-ductive number of SARS-CoV-2 was initially 14.8—four times higher than in Wuhan, China, the original epicenter of the COVID-19 pandemic.[27] This means that, on average, each Di-amond Princess passenger infected with SARS-CoV-2 spread the virus to almost 15 other people (refer to Chapter 1, "Coron-avirus: Basics and Background," for a more detailed discussion of the basic reproductive number or R_0).

Cruise ships foster outbreaks of disease due to a number of factors: infectious diseases spread rapidly due to a large number of people confined to a relatively small space, passen-gers from diverse regions intermingle over the course of six to seven days—which is long enough for people in the incu-bation period to become symptomatic, and outbreaks can be sustained by crew members who remain onboard for multiple trips.[28,29]

In addition to the increased risk of infectious disease, a cruise ship is not the best place to fall ill. Medical care aboard cruise ships varies by ship size, itinerary, length of cruise, and passenger demographics.[30] While medical care on board cruise ships is usually comparable to that of an ambulatory care center, cruise ships are not hospitals, so passengers may face limitations in care due to a lack of medical capabilities and supplies.

Is it okay to leave hand sanitizer in my car?

The simple answer is yes; you can leave hand sanitizer in your car. However, you should avoid doing so during the summer and winter months. Hand sanitizer should not be stored in freezing temperatures or above 105° F (40° C)[31]; it is best kept at temperatures between 59 - 86° F (15 - 30° C). Additionally, alcohol-based hand sanitizer is poisonous and should not be ingested—if left in the car, make sure it remains out of children's reach.[32]

References

1. Centers for Disease Control and Prevention. Considerations for travelers - coronavirus in the US. Centers for Disease Control and Prevention. https://www.cdc.gov/coronavirus/2019-ncov/travelers/travel-in-the-us.html. Published 2020. Accessed 2020.

2. Fauver JR, Petrone ME, Hodcroft EB, et al. Coast-to-coast spread of SARS-CoV-2 during the early epidemic in the United States. *Cell.* 2020.

3. Governor Press Office. Tri-State advisory will use uniform parameters and messaging across the three states effective midnight tonight. https://www.governor.ny.gov/news/governor-cuomo-governor-murphy-and-governor-lamont-announce-joint-incoming-travel-advisory-all. Published June 24 2020. Accessed 2020.

4. Centers for Disease Control and Prevention. How COVID-19 spreads. Centers for Disease Control and Prevention. https://www.cdc.gov/coronavirus/

2019-ncov/prevent-getting-sick/how-covid-spreads.html. Published June 1, 2020.

5. McKeever A. Here's how coronavirus spreads on a plane—and the safest place to sit. *National Geographic.* 2020. https://www.nationalgeographic.com/science/2020/01/how-coronavirus-spreads-on-a-plane/. Published March 6 2020.

6. Hertzberg VS, Weiss H, Elon L, Si W, Norris SL, Fly. Healthy Research T. Behaviors, movements, and transmission of droplet-mediated respiratory diseases during transcontinental airline flights. *Proceedings of the National Academy of Sciences of the United States of America.* 2018;115(14):3623-3627.

7. Centers for Disease Control and Prevention. Considerations for travelers - Coronavirus in the US. https://www.cdc.gov/coronavirus/2019-ncov/travelers/travel-in-the-us.html. Published May 28 2020. Accessed 2020.

8. Transportation Security Administration. Hand sanitizers. US Department of Homeland Security. https://www.tsa.gov/travel/security-screening/whatcanibring/items/hand-sanitizers. Published 2020.

9. Peterson B, Dunn D. Is it safe to travel again? Your coronavirus questions answered. *Wall Street Journal.* 2020. https://www.wsj.com/articles/all-your-coronavirus-travel-questions-answered-11582980999. Published June 10 2020.

10. Doucleff M, Huang P. How not to get sick on a plane: A guide to avoiding pathogens. National Public Radio. The Corona Crisis Web site. https://www.npr.org/sec-

tions/goatsandsoda/2020/02/13/804860215/how-not-to-get-sick-on-a-plane-a-guide-to-avoiding-pathogens. Published 2020. Accessed 2020.

11. Mangili A, Vindenes T, Gendreau M. Infectious risks of air travel. *Microbiology Spectrum*. 2015;3(5).

12. Martinez L, Blanc L, Nunn P, Raviglione M. Tuberculosis and air travel: WHO guidance in the era of drug-resistant TB. *Travel Med Infect Dis*. 2008;6(4):177-181.

13. International Air Transport Association. Cabin air quality – Risk of communicable diseases transmission. Montreal. January 2018.

14. O'Sullivan F. In Japan and France, riding transit looks surprisingly safe. *CityLab* 2020.

15. Centers for Disease Control and Prevention. Protect yourself when using transportation. https://www.cdc.gov/coronavirus/2019-ncov/daily-life-coping/using-transportation.html#TypesofTransportation. Published 2020. Accessed 2020.

16. Quilty BJ, Clifford S, Flasche S, Eggo RM. Effectiveness of airport screening at detecting travellers infected with novel coronavirus (2019-nCoV). *Euro Surveill*. 2020;25(5).

17. Mbala P, Baguelin M, Ngay I, et al. Evaluating the frequency of asymptomatic Ebola virus infection. *Philos Trans R Soc Lond B Biol Sci*. 2017;372(1721).

18. Centers for Disease Control and Prevention. Before you travel tips. https://wwwnc.cdc.gov/travel/page/before-travel. Published September 23 2019. Accessed 2020.

19. World Health Organization. Management of ill travellers at points of entry – international airports, ports and ground crossings – in the context of the COVID-19 outbreak. World Health Organization;March 19 2020.

20. Affairs UDoS-BoC. Travel Advisories. US Department of State. https://travel.state.gov/content/travel/en/traveladvisories/traveladvisories.html/. Published 2020. Accessed 2020.

21. Salcedo A, Yar S, Cherelus G. Coronavirus travel restrictions, across the globe. *The New York Times.* Published July 16 2020.

22. Hardingham-Gill T. Which international destinations are reopening to tourists? Cable News Network. https://www.cnn.com/travel/article/global-destinations-reopening-to-tourists/index.html. Published 2020. Accessed 2020.

23. U.S. Department of State. COVID-19 Traveler Information. Bureau of Consular Affairs. https://travel.state.gov/content/travel/en/traveladvisories/ea/covid-19-information.html. Published 2020. Accessed 2020.

24. U.S. Department of State. Smart Traveler Enrollment Program. Bureau of Consular Affairs. https://step.state.gov. Accessed 2020.

25. U.S. Centers for Medicare & Medicaid Services. Travel Medical Coverage. U.S. Centers for Medicare & Medicaid Services. https://www.medicare.gov/coverage/travel. Accessed 2020.

26. Centers for Disease Control and Prevention. COVID-19 and Cruise Ship Travel. https://www.nc.cdc.gov/travel/notices/warning/coronavirus-cruise-ship. Published April 20 2020. Accessed 2020.

27. Rocklöv J, Sjödin H, Wilder-Smith A. COVID-19 outbreak on the Diamond Princess cruise ship: estimating the epidemic potential and effectiveness of public health countermeasures. *J Travel Med.* 2020;27(3).

28. Kak V. Infections on Cruise Ships. *Microbiology Spectrum.* 2015;3(4).

29. Pavli A, Maltezou HC, Papadakis A, et al. Respiratory infections and gastrointestinal illness on a cruise ship: A three-year prospective study. *Travel Medicine and Infectious Disease.* 2016;14(4):389-397.

30. Centers for Disease Control and Prevention. Cruise Ship Travel. In: *CDC Yellow Book 2020: Health Information for International Travel.* New York: Oxford University Press; 2020.

31. US Food and Drug Administration. Q&A for consumers: Hand Sanitizers and COVID-19. https://www.fda.gov/drugs/information-drug-class/qa-consumers-hand-sanitizers-and-covid-19. Published June 06 2020. Accessed 2020.

32. U.S. Food and Drug Administration. Safely using hand sanitizer. https://www.fda.gov/consumers/consumer-updates/safely-using-hand-sanitizer. Published March 30 2020. Accessed 2020.

FOR HEALTHCARE WORKERS

What changes can be made to the work environment to prevent transmission?

Depending on the work environment (e.g., clinic, hospital, office), many precautions can be put in place to prevent the spread of COVID-19.

The virus SARS-CoV-2 spreads through respiratory droplets, so the best way to prevent transmission is to reduce in-person visits when possible. Quality healthcare can still be provided through telemedicine—communication between physician and patient through live chat, phone calls, and video conferences.[1] Telemedicine allows patients to stay at home while still being able to interact with their physician, ask questions, get expert advice, and have prescriptions sent to their local pharmacies.[1] By preventing the physical patient visit to a clinic or hospital, telemedicine can prevent virus transmission without compromising patient care.[1]

One of the shortcomings of telemedicine, however, is the inability to physically examine the patient. While some visits, like those for prescription refills or regular chronic disease follow-ups, can often forgo a physical exam, other visits—such as those for abdominal pain or pap smears—cannot.[1] If a physical exam is necessary, patients should be encouraged to see their doctor in person, and appropriate measures should be put in place on both sides to ensure a safe and productive visit.[1]

· **The waiting area**

One of the easiest ways to prevent the spread of the virus in waiting areas is to provide the proper supplies for people using that space. Waiting rooms should include masks, alcohol-based hand sanitizers, tissues, and trash cans, all of which should be easily visible and accessible.[2] All seating spaces in the waiting room should be kept at least 6 feet apart whenever possible, and glass screens can be placed in between the front desk and waiting area to add an extra layer of protection to employees behind the desk.[3]

Minimize overcrowding in the waiting room by encouraging patients to stay in their cars until they can be seen, and ask anyone accompanying the patient to stay in the car during the patient's entire visit if possible.[2,4] For some clinics, having patients wait in their vehicles may allow the waiting area to be done away with entirely. Upon entering the waiting area, each patient's temperature should be checked, and everyone—patients, physicians, and clinical staff—should be wearing masks properly at all times.[3] If a patient has a fever, the patient should be removed from any common areas and allowed to wait in a designated exam room for symptomatic patients. If no such rooms are available and climate permits, the patient can be asked to wait outside to prevent exposure to other patients and staff. If the waiting area usually has toys, magazines, or other communal objects, these should either be removed or cleaned regularly to prevent possible contamination.[2]

· **The exam room**

A typical clinic exam room is small, which allows SARS-CoV-2 to spread easily if proper precautions are not taken. Only the patient and medical worker should be in the exam room whenever possible; anyone accompanying the patient should be asked to wait outside to maximize the physical distance possible within the room.[2,4] Inside the room, both the healthcare worker and patient should wear masks at all times and attempt to sit at least 6 feet apart.[4]

While physical contact should be minimized, the quality of physical exams should not suffer, and healthcare workers can perform a thorough exam with safety precautions in place. During physical exams, gloves should be worn by the medical worker, masks should be tightly secured around the mouth and nose of both the patient and medical professional, and talking should be minimized.[3] After the physical exam is complete, physical distancing of at least 6 feet should be resumed.[4]

If healthcare workers expect to come in close contact with bodily fluids, they should wear a face shield in addition to their regular protective gear.[5] Face shields offer an extra layer of protection that covers all areas of the face that are potential virus entry points (eyes, nose, mouth) and are necessary when dealing with spraying or splattering body fluids.[5] Face shields should always be used as an adjunct to other personal protective equipment (PPE); they are not suitable to use as solitary facial protection due to their inability to form a peripheral seal.

For visits with low to zero potential exposure to bodily fluids, face shields or goggles are still recommended—however, adherence to this practice varies widely by geographic region and hospital system.[5]

After the patient leaves, the most frequently used and touched areas of the room (e.g., counters, exam table, chairs, computers) should be wiped down using EPA-registered disinfectants.[6]

· **The operating room**

Patients should delay non-emergent surgeries in order to avoid being at the hospital while COVID-19 is prevalent.[7] If the patient is unable to delay surgery, they should undergo a reverse transcriptase–polymerase chain reaction (RT-PCR) test to determine if they are carrying the virus.[7] If the patient tests positive, all medical staff present in the operating room during the surgery must wear an N95 mask.[7] If the patient tests negative and has no history of fever, COVID-19 symptoms, or exposure to SARS-CoV-2, the surgical team can proceed with the surgery as usual (i.e., regular surgical masks instead of N95s) without additional precautions.[7]

Staff who are performing intubations, extensive bag mask ventilation, or aerosol-generating procedures should wear an N95 mask and a face shield during the entire procedure.[7] In addition, during any procedure that requires the patient's mouth to be open for an extended period of time, personnel who are not immediately necessary should not be present.[7]

Operating rooms are generally very thoroughly disinfected. During the COVID-19 era, staff disinfecting the OR should follow usual cleaning procedures while following droplet precautions, which requires wearing surgical masks.[7]

· **Non-patient areas and offices**

Anyone who does not have to be physically present at the hospital or clinic should be encouraged to work and attend meetings from home.[6] Those who cannot work from home should have their temperature checked daily as they enter and should go home if their temperature is elevated or they are experiencing cough, shortness of breath, or fatigue.[4]

Everyone should wear a mask at all times and wash their hands frequently.[2] Dividing patient areas from non-patient areas with plastic or glass partitions will allow for easy communication while potentially preventing the spread of respiratory droplets between both sides of the divider.[3] At the end of the day, offices and non-patient areas should be thoroughly disinfected with EPA-registered disinfectants.[6]

Nonclinical areas and offices can follow many of the precautions discussed in Chapter 5: "Work, School, and the Office".

Should all patients wear masks?

Regardless of whether patients feel sick, they should wear masks when visiting a doctor's office or hospital.[8] Wearing a mask prevents the patient's own respiratory droplets from spreading to others and also protects the patient from exposure to others' respiratory droplets.[8] In addition, wearing a mask prevents the patient from accidentally touching their face and potentially exposing their nose or mouth to the virus or other contaminants.[8]

While there are some instances in which wearing a mask does more harm than good—for example, in severe trigeminal neuralgia, during zoster reactivation, or after facial surgery—these are rare and should be considered on a case-by-case basis. Patients with mild breathing problems such as well-controlled asthma or COPD should wear masks.[8] Patients with difficulty breathing are encouraged to speak with their physician about their individual risk and proceed based on the medical advice they receive.[8]

It may be difficult to enforce mask-wearing in the pediatric population.[8] Young children may not want to wear masks due to discomfort, and while some may have a vague idea of the COVID pandemic, many do not have a concrete understanding of what is going on or why masks are so important.[8] Parents are encouraged to speak with their children about the importance of wearing a mask when visiting the doctor and to take time to answer questions their child has about the pandemic.[8] While older children will likely understand the importance of wearing a mask, younger children may refuse to wear one.[8] In this case, parents must be extra vigilant about distancing from others, attending to what their child is touching in public areas (not only the doctor's office or hospital), and if they are touching their face frequently.[8] Parents should encourage their children to wash their hands or use hand sanitizer regularly when outside the home.[8]

Wearing a mask can be uncomfortable, but it plays a vital role in preventing the spread of COVID-19. All patients should wear masks except children under the age of two, those with severe respiratory conditions who have been advised against masks by their physician, and those who are unable to remove their masks independently.[8]

Should patients come in for routine outpatient care?

Routine outpatient care is usually not an emergency; therefore, patients should be encouraged to see their doctor from home through telemedicine whenever possible.[6] For visits that require physical interaction (e.g., lab work, Pap smears), consider the likelihood of harm if care is deferred.[9] If community transmission is high and care can be safely postponed, defer the visit. Otherwise, the visit can be scheduled as usual with safety precautions in place.

How can I protect my family and other close contacts?

This is one of the most important and frequently asked questions by healthcare workers in the COVID-19 era. One of the best ways healthcare workers can protect their loved ones is by taking proper precautions at work.[6] While donning extra protective gear and wearing masks all day may be uncomfortable, these practices are necessary to ensure that workers and their loved ones are protected at home.[6]

Health care workers should wash their hands regularly and thoroughly as well as make a conscious effort to not touch their faces.[4] In addition, healthcare workers should consider immediately changing clothes before entering their homes to add an extra layer of protection between their family and potentially contaminated work clothing.[4]

Many healthcare professionals are choosing to protect their loved ones by physically living apart from them for an extended period. While this may be a safe option, it can also be damaging to the mental well-being of both the healthcare workers and their families.[10] Spiking cases of COVID-19 have forced health professionals to work overtime, experience more fatigue than usual, and face the emotional toll that comes with patient deaths.[10] These factors are unique to healthcare and take a great toll on mental health; during stressful times healthcare workers need support more than ever.[10] Therefore, healthcare workers are encouraged to take precautions while at work, when leaving work, and before entering their homes to balance the physical safety of their loved ones with mental peace for themselves.[10]

- **Specific practices healthcare workers can take to protect their loved ones[11]:**
  -Frequent hand washing
  -Avoid unnecessary accessories (e.g., jewelry)
  -Put long hair up in a bun or braid, or cover up hair completely if possible (e.g., wear a scrub cap)

-Strictly adhere to PPE recommendations

-Change out of work clothes before entering the home

-Sanitize every-day items after returning home (e.g., cell phone, car keys)

-Shower immediately after returning home

-Dedicate a set of eating utensils specifically for the medical worker and wash them with soap and water immediately after use

-Avoid touching food that others will eat

-Dedicate a separate bathroom specifically for the medical worker

-Get tested for COVID-19 frequently if possible

Which workers are highest risk?

Members of the healthcare field are at highest risk, with members of the dental field (e.g., dental hygienists, dental assistants, and dentists) having the highest risk of all.[10] Patients spend a large portion of time at the dentist's office with their mouths open, which allows respiratory droplets to spread easily.[10] After members of the dental field, the next highest risk groups are general practitioners and nurses who are usually the first to see a patient when they feel sick.[10]

Anesthesiologists, emergency physicians, and nurse anesthetists have also been reported to be at high risk for COVID-19. However, this claim is anecdotal and no studies examining these professions' risk have been performed.

Can masks be safely re-used?

While it is easier, safer, and cleaner to not re-use masks, sometimes it is necessary to re-use them due to low supply.

Masks can be safely reused if the proper precautions are taken to sanitize them.[12]

If I have to re-use a mask, what is the best way to sterilize or decontaminate it?

If a mask must be re-used, it must be decontaminated to prevent viral particles from infecting the wearer with subsequent uses. The proper way to decontaminate a mask depends on the type of mask and its material content.[12]

Used surgical masks that are not visibly soiled can be stored in a container in a designated decontamination area for 72 hours before being used again.[12] The container should not be air-tight, as air flow helps with drying and may help inactivate the virus.[12] The 72-hour period is long enough to inactivate any SARS-CoV-2 particles that may be on the mask's surface.

Surgical masks should be worn in clinical settings due to their ability to provide both mechanical and electrostatic filtration (refer to Chapter 2, "General Safety," for more detailed information on mask types). In nonclinical settings, however, cloth masks may be adequate. Cloth masks can be treated like most other pieces of clothing and laundered in a washer and dryer.[12] They do not need to be separated from other clothing, but they should be washed after each use to ensure they are clean and safe to wear again.[12] If a washing machine is not available, handwashing the mask with hot water and detergent and allowing it to air dry in a clean environment is also a viable solution.[12] Over time and multiple washings, the fabric of cloth masks can wear thin which offers less protection; therefore, it is important to remain aware of the status of the cloth mask and replace it if needed.[12]

In March and April—early in the pandemic—N95 masks were in very short supply. As of August 2020, the supply chain appears to have improved, although the CDC still recommends conserving N95 masks for healthcare workers.[12] While effective methods for N95 sterilization are still being explored, four methods currently in use include exposing the used mask to ultraviolet light, 70% ethanol spray, temperatures greater than 158°F (70°C), or vaporized hydrogen peroxide.[12] While these methods are effective, they are not without risk; ethanol spray, for example, damages the fit of the mask and makes it unusable after two sessions of disinfection. UV light and heat produce the same result after three sessions.[12] Vaporized hydrogen peroxide is more effective than the other methods at both sanitizing the mask and preserving its usable life.[12]

What are some reusable PPE options?

Ideally, healthcare workers would use new PPE for every patient encounter; however, a nationwide shortage of PPE may make reusable options a necessity.

Elastomeric respirators and Powered Air Purifying Respirators (PAPR) can be used instead of disposable masks if they are available. These respirators effectively protect against respiratory droplets and aerosols, and they can be easily cleaned with soap and water solutions.[13] Elastomeric respirators are used almost exclusively at the Texas Center for Infectious Disease (TCID), a small hospital which exclusively treats patients with tuberculosis. No TCID staff have tested positive for tuberculosis since 1994 (elastomeric respirators were introduced in 1995).[13]

Although less critical than respiratory protection, face shields, goggles, and cloth isolation gowns are all reusable as well. Face shields and goggles can be thoroughly wiped both on the inside and outside before being reused, and cloth isolation gowns can be laundered on-site.[14] However, widespread shortages of these types of PPE have not been reported.

Caring properly for reusable PPE will extend its usable lifetime, and medical workers should be vigilant about identifying worn out equipment that puts themselves and patients at risk.[14] Worn out PPE should be thrown away and replaced as soon as possible.[14]

What should I look for when purchasing N95 respirators?

In a healthcare setting, PPE will typically be provided. However, if it is not, individuals looking to purchase N95 respirators should be wary of purchasing counterfeit respirators. The National Institute for Occupational Safety and Health (NIOSH) is responsible for regulating and approving N95 respirators, and counterfeit respirators will not meet the filtering standards required for N95 designation.

The CDC has reported increasing sales and production of counterfeit N95 masks during the COVID-19 pandemic and produced a guide to help consumers avoid counterfeit products.

- **NIOSH-approved N95s will have the following markings:**
  -NIOSH approval on the respirator packaging or contents
  -An abbreviated approval on the portion of the mask

that covers the face[15]

- **The following indicators suggest that an N95 is counterfeit:**
  -No markings or approvals on the portion of the mask that covers the face
  -No approval numbers on the mask or elastic band
  -"NIOSH" spelled incorrectly
  -Any decorative fabric or trim on the respirator
  -Any claims of approval for children—NIOSH does not approve any form of respiratory PPE for children
  -Masks with ear loops instead of elastic head-band—ear loops typically do not form a tight enough seal between the mask and face to meet N95 requirements[15]

The CDC has posted numerous examples of counterfeit N95 respirators online (www.cdc.gov/niosh/npptl/user-notices/counterfeitResp.html) which may be helpful when discerning real from fake N95s. If at all possible, avoid purchasing PPE from third-party sellers and drop shipping companies.

References

1. Alvandi M. Telemedicine and its role in revolutionizing healthcare delivery. *Am J Accountable Care.* 2017;5: e1-e5. https://www.ajmc.com/journals/ajac/2017/2017-vol5-n1/telemedicine-and-its-role-in-revolutionizing-healthcare-delivery.

2. Centers for Disease Control and Prevention. Coronavirus (COVID-19) workplace tips for employees. https://www.cdc.gov/coronavirus/2019-ncov/community/guidance-business-response.html. Published 2020.

3. U.S. Department of Labor: Occupational Safety and Health Administration. Guidance on preparing workplaces for COVID-19. OSHA. 2020:35.

4. The Lancet. COVID-19: protecting health-care workers. 2020;395(10228):922. Published March 21, 2020.

5. Roberge RJ. Face shields for infection control: A review. *J Occup Environ Hyg.* 2016;13(4):239-246.

6. Delgado D, Quintana FW, Perez G, et al. Personal safety during the covid-19 pandemic: Realities and perspectives of healthcare workers in latin America. *Int J Environ Res Public Health.* 2020;17(8):1-8.

7. Forrester JD, Nassar AK, Maggio PM, Hawn MT. Precautions for operating room team members during the COVID-19 pandemic. *J Am Coll Surg.* 2020;230(6):1098-1101.

8. Centers for Disease Control and Prevention. Coronavirus Disease 2019 (COVID-19) considerations for wearing cloth face coverings: evidence for effectiveness of cloth face coverings. https://www.cdc.gov/coronavirus/2019-ncov/prevent-getting-sick/cloth-face-cover-guidance.html. Published 2020.

9. Centers for Disease Control and Prevention. Framework for Healthcare Systems Providing Non-COVID-19 Clinical Care During the COVID-19 Pandemic. https://www.cdc.gov/coronavirus/2019-ncov/

hcp/framework-non-COVID-care.html. Published
2020.

10. World Health Organization. Coronavirus Disease
(Covid-19) Outbreak: Rights, roles and responsibilities
of health workers, including key considerations for
occupational safety. World Heal Organ.
2020;(March):1-3.

11. Harris CA, Evan HL, Telem DA. A Practical Decontamination Framework for COVID-19 Front-line Workers
Returning Home [published online ahead of print,
2020 May 1]. *Ann Surg.* 2020;10.1097/
SLA.0000000000003990.

12. U.S. Department of Labor: Occupational Safety and
Health Administration. Prevent Worker Exposure to
Coronavirus (COVID-19). OSHA. (6742):6742.

13. National Academies of Sciences, Engineering, and
Medicine. 2019. *Reusable Elastomeric Respirators in
Health Care: Considerations for Routine and Surge Use.*
Washington, DC: The National Academies Press.
https://doi.org/10.17226/25275

14. Joint Commission. How to reuse PPE masks & N95
respirators. How to clean eye protection equipment.
How to remove a gown for reuse. https://www.joint-
commission.org/covid-19/. Published 2020.

15. Centers for Disease Control and Prevention. Counterfeit Respirators / Misrepresentation of NIOSH-Ap-
proval. https://www.cdc.gov/niosh/npptl/usernotices/
counterfeitResp.html. Accessed August 2020.

EXPOSURE TO COVID-19, TESTING, AND ILLNESS

How long does it take to develop symptoms of COVID-19?

It can take anywhere from 2 to 14 days for symptoms of COVID-19 to appear; however, most people will develop symptoms within five days of exposure.[1] Symptoms may include fever, cough, sore throat, fatigue, headache, and breathlessness.

Can I infect other people if I have no symptoms?

There are two groups of people who do not show symptoms: asymptomatic people (those who never develop symptoms) and pre-symptomatic people (those who yield positive test results for SARS-CoV-2 before symptoms develop).[2] There may be a window period in which an individual is infectious yet has not developed symptoms. It is difficult to classify individuals as asymptomatic or pre-symptomatic; patients first classified as asymptomatic during testing may later be reclassified as having been pre-symptomatic when symptoms develop.[2]

Pre-symptomatic people can transmit the virus prior to symptom onset. A Chinese study on viral loads found that up to 44% of patients had transmitted SARS-CoV-2 to other patients two to three days before symptom onset.[2] In Singapore, a study of 157 people found that 10 secondary cases were most likely acquired before symptoms developed in the initial cases. In another study, an asymptomatic patient had a viral load comparable to symptomatic patients, suggesting that SARS-CoV-2 can be transmitted by people who never develop symptoms.[3]

However, little is known about asymptomatic viral transmission other than it is possible, so it is best to be cautious and behave as though asymptomatic people are potentially infectious.

I was exposed to SARS-CoV-2 and now have mild symptoms. Should I stay home or get tested?

If you think you have been exposed to SARS-CoV-2 and have developed symptoms of COVID-19, contact a physician. If you have been experiencing fever, cough, or any other COVID-19-related symptoms, your physician will most likely order a lab test for you. This test will determine if you have contracted the virus and need to self-isolate.

Most individuals can recover at home if the illness is mild. If your symptoms are more urgent—such as difficulty breathing—seek emergency assistance immediately. Do not leave your home unless advised to do so by your physician.[4] Do not visit public establishments or use public transportation.

How does testing for COVID-19 work?

Testing for COVID-19 requires an order from a physician. There are two types of test available: a viral swab test and a saliva-based test. For the viral swab test, a nasal or throat swab is inserted deep into the nose or throat. This is often uncomfortable for the patient. The swab is kept in the nose for at least ten seconds and twisted around three times.[5] The specimen is then sent to a laboratory and results are typically available within a week.

The saliva-based test is less invasive since the person being tested needs only to be able to spit into a cup. This form of testing is more comfortable for the person being tested, and it requires less personal protective equipment than the swab test because it involves little interaction with healthcare workers.[6]

Both types of tests look for SARS-CoV-2 genetic material, and both tests are very reliable when positive.[6] If someone tests positive, the likelihood of their having the virus is high. However, if someone tests negative, there is still a possibility that they are infected.

If I test positive but have no symptoms, should I self-quarantine?

The Centers for Disease Control and Prevention (CDC) recommends self-quarantine if you have been exposed to the virus or have tested positive for the virus. Self-quarantine should last a total of 14 days, starting from the last day of exposure to someone infected with SARS-CoV-2. Do not leave your home unless necessary and avoid contact with other people who live in your home. Refrain from contact with animals. Perform meticulous hand washing to prevent spread. Do not share bedding, towels, dishes, utensils, or drinks with other people. Disinfect phones, bathroom, counters, and keyboards every day. Be aware of your symptoms and check your temperature daily.

Who should get tested?

According to the CDC, viral testing should be performed in individuals who show signs and symptoms of COVID-19, those who are asymptomatic but have been exposed to the virus, and those who are asymptomatic but work in a high-risk setting.[7] Since both asymptomatic and pre-symptomatic transmission are possible, it is imperative to test individuals who have been exposed to SARS-CoV-2 to rapidly identify infected individuals.[7] The more rapidly someone is identified as SARS-CoV-2-positive, the sooner they can start self-isolation and the sooner contact tracing can begin, reducing the amount of time during which they may unknowingly infect others.

Testing is also recommended in community, outpatient, and hospital-based surveillance systems to identify disease trends and predict potential impacts on communities over time.[7]

What is a false negative? How likely is it?

A false negative is "a test result that indicates that a person does not have a specific disease or condition when the person actually does have the disease or condition."[8] The false-negative rate for COVID-19 viral swab testing depends upon the number of days after exposure.

In a study evaluating 1,330 viral swab samples, false-negative rates decreased from 100% on day 1 to 67% on day 4.[9] This means that one day after exposure to SARS-CoV-2 the test will be negative regardless of whether the person contracted the virus. This may be attributed to a viral load beneath the detectable range as well as improper technique or handling of the specimen. On day 8, approximately three days after the onset of symptoms, the chance of a false-negative test drops to 21%.[9] It is not clear whether this number will drop any lower. Therefore, ruling out SARS-CoV-2 infection based only on viral testing should be used with caution. Additionally, nursing homes are being selective about admitting patients from hospitals due to the possibility of false-negative results. Some facilities are demanding two different tests showing negative results before accepting a patient.[10]

Why do some people get sicker than others?

For some people, COVID-19 presents as a mild upper respiratory illness, while other people become extremely ill and require admission to a hospital's intensive care unit. According to Dr. Aiko Iwasake, a Yale immunobiologist, this variability in presentation of symptoms can be attributed to whether people experience "cytokine storm," which is an overactivation of the body's immune response.[11] When the virus infects an individual, the body responds by secreting immune signals called cytokines which recruit immune cells that help fight the virus. However, in some individuals, too many cytokines are produced. The immune system responds by attacking normal, healthy tissue, which leads to the breakdown of linings that protect the lungs and blood vessels. This can worsen existing symptoms and cause additional problems such as difficulty breathing, high fever, kidney failure, and possibly death. Cytokine storm is more likely to occur in people over the age of 60, smokers, and those with chronic lung disease, immuno-suppression, or cancer.[12]

How long will it take to recover?

According to the World Health Organization, recovery ranges from two to six weeks. For people with mild cases, recovery time is typically two weeks. More severe illness can cause the recovery period to last up to six weeks.[13] Recovery in individuals varies but usually involves resolution of aches, fever, and cough. It is possible to be contagious for up to a week once symptoms have resolved.[14]

What is the recovery rate?

Recovery rate is the number of recovered cases divided by the number of total cases (both recovered and deceased). If someone is asymptomatic, they can be considered recovered once they clear the virus. If someone clears the virus but sustains permanent lung damage, they are still considered recovered.[15] People are typically considered recovered from COVID-19 when symptoms and fever have resolved; recovery can also be confirmed with two negative test results.

It is nearly impossible to give an accurate measurement of the recovery rate for COVID-19. Recovery rates may be underestimated due to asymptomatic patients and lack of testing. Many sources claim that the recovery rate is 98%, but this has not been verified by the CDC or any reputable source. The mortality rate worldwide is about 1%. Dr. Anthony Fauci, director of the National Institute of Allergy and Infectious Diseases, simplifies what this means: with a mortality rate of 1%, COVID-19 is "10-times more lethal than the seasonal flu."[16] Fatality rates also vary by age: children younger than 10 years old have a case fatality rate of almost 0%, individuals 10 to 50 years old have a fatality rate of less than 1%, while the elderly population (those over 60 years old) are at highest risk with a case fatality rate up to 20%.[17]

What does it mean to self-isolate? Is self-isolation different from quarantine?

Self-isolation is the separation of people infected with the virus (both symptomatic and asymptomatic individuals) from people who are not infected with the virus.[18] Quarantine separates people who have been exposed to the virus to see if they become sick. Both require an individual to stay at home until it is safe for them to be around other people. Staying at home for a minimum of 14 days after your last exposure is recommended. If you do need to leave your home, practice social distancing and wear a mask.

Can I self-isolate in a shared house?

Yes, it is possible to self-isolate in a shared house. Try to avoid other people and animals (e.g., pets). Stay in one specific room or area that is not used by other people in the shared house. Use a separate bathroom if possible.[18]

If I develop COVID-19, will I also develop immunity to it? Can I get re-infected?

According to the World Health Organization, "there is currently no evidence that people who have recovered from COVID-19 and have antibodies are protected from a second infection."[19] Because we are not certain whether infection provides immunity, it is best to err on the side of caution and behave as though re-infection is possible. People who assume that they are immune from contracting COVID-19 a second time may opt to ignore public health guidelines and thus contribute to increased risk of transmission.

If I develop immunity, how long will it last?

At this time, there is no substantial evidence that supports the development of immunity against SARS-CoV-2.[19] If immunity does develop, it is not yet possible to say how long it will last.

Are there any lingering after-effects in people who recover?

Dr. Aaron Glatt, the chief of infectious diseases at Mount Sinai South Nassau, explains that during recovery from COVID-19 it is common to feel symptoms of malaise, low tolerance to exercise, and weakness.[20] Additionally, even after lung function has returned to normal, it is not uncommon to experience periods of shortness of breath.

Dr. Joseph Coniglaro, the chief of general internal medicine at Northwell Health in New York, has also witnessed a multitude of lingering after-effects in people who have recovered from severe illness. These effects include, but are not limited to, organs involving the kidneys, gastrointestinal tract, and nervous system.[20] COVID-19 has the potential to cause acute kidney injury, which reduces the body's ability to filter waste from the blood and produce urine. Gastrointestinal effects include diarrhea, nausea, vomiting, and abdominal pain.[21] Neurological complications such as difficulty with balancing and walking, seizures, nerve pain, and stroke may also occur.[22] It is not clear if these effects are permanent since there is minimal long-term data. After recovery, this variety of lingering symptoms can be attributed to the inflammatory response of the body; they are not necessarily due to the virus itself.

The psychological impact of COVID-19 varies from person to person. However, since the outbreak, people have reported increased feelings of stress, fear, and anxiety regarding the uncertainty of this disease.[23]

What is an antibody test? How accurate is it?

Antibody testing looks for the presence of small proteins circulating in the blood that indicate whether a person has been infected by a pathogen (typically a virus or bacterium). Antibodies are an important part of the immune system and serve to block pathogens from infecting other cells or flag them for destruction by other immune cells. Antibodies start forming one to three weeks after infection.[24]

Antibody testing is performed after full recovery from a disease and is used to determine whether an individual has antibodies against the virus or bacteria that caused the disease.[25] Testing requires a blood sample, which can be obtained through a finger prick or a blood draw from a vein. If the test results show SARS-CoV-2 antibodies, this confirms that you were once infected with the virus and may have some amount of immunity against it.[25] However, the WHO has stated that there is a lack of evidence about protection against re-infection.[19]

The accuracy of the test is highly dependent on the time the test is performed. There is also the possibility of cross-reactivity, meaning antibodies from other coronaviruses (e.g., common cold) can be identified. If blood is drawn early in the course of infection, antibodies are less likely to be present. Therefore, antibody tests should be performed after an individual has fully recovered from the illness. Given these limitations, antibody tests are not completely accurate and should not be used alone to diagnose COVID-19.

Can COVID-19 cause permanent damage to my lungs or other organs?

Yes, COVID-19 can cause permanent damage to a person's lungs. This damage is mediated by the body's inflammatory response to SARS-CoV-2. Mild cases of COVID-19 have a much lower chance of causing severe, long-lasting lung damage compared with severe cases.[26] If scarring of the lung occurs, it can take months to years for full recovery to occur. In some cases, the damage is irreparable (one woman in Chicago suffered irreversible damage to her lungs and required a double lung transplant).

COVID-19 does have the ability to affect other organs in addition to the lungs. The International Society of Nephrology states that roughly a quarter of patients who require hospitalization for COVID-19 develop some sort of kidney problem.[27] Additionally, the American Neurological Association states that about a third of patients hospitalized with COVID-19 acquire neurological symptoms, such as dizziness, headaches, strokes, and shifts in consciousness.[27] Many people who have developed damage to multiple organs were hospitalized and had contracted a severe form of the illness.

Does COVID-19 have any effect on the heart?

Yes, COVID-19 can affect the heart. Individuals with preexisting heart conditions (e.g., heart attack, atherosclerosis) have a higher chance of developing a severe cardiac complication from the virus compared with patients without pre-existing conditions. Some people have also experienced symptoms that mimic a heart attack even if they do not have fatty plaques in their arteries (this is often the cause of typical heart attacks).[28]

COVID-19 can also affect people without pre-existing heart conditions and cause inflammation of the heart tissue. This can lead to abnormal heart rhythms and the inability to properly pump blood throughout the body.[28] These complications can range from mild to severe. Severe complications are rare, but possible.

Are there medications I should avoid if I catch COVID-19?

Currently, there is no evidence that taking anti-inflammatory medications (e.g., naproxen, ibuprofen) can exacerbate COVID-19.[29] Drugs such as acetaminophen, naproxen, or ibuprofen can be used to reduce fever and manage pain and muscle aches. Any changes to current medications, such as blood pressure medication or immunosuppressants, should be made by your physician only.

References

1. Singhal T. A Review of Coronavirus Disease-2019 (COVID-19). *Indian J Pediatr.* 2020;87(4):281-286.
2. Lee S, Meyler P, Mozel M, Tauh T, Merchant R. Asymptomatic carriage and transmission of SARS-CoV-2: What do we know? *Can J Anaesth.* 2020.

3. Gao Z, Xu Y, Sun C, et al. A Systematic review of asymptomatic infections with COVID-19. *J Microbiol Immunol Infect.* 2020.

4. Centers for Disease Control and Prevention. What to Do If You Are Sick. https://www.cdc.gov/coronavirus/2019-ncov/if-you-are-sick/steps-when-sick.html. Published 2020.

5. Tang Y-W, Schmitz JE, Persing DH, Stratton CW. Laboratory diagnosis of COVID-19: Current issues and challenges. *Journal of Clinical Microbiology.* 2020;58(6):e00512-00520.

6. School HM. If you've been exposed to the coronavirus. *Harvard Health Publishing.* 2020.

7. Centers for Disease Control and Prevention. Overview of Testing for SARS-CoV-2. https://www.cdc.gov/coronavirus/2019-ncov/hcp/testing-overview.html. Published 2020.

8. National Institutes of Health: National Cancer Institute. NCI Dictionary. https://www.cancer.gov/publications/dictionaries/cancer-terms/.

9. Kucirka LM, Lauer SA, Laeyendecker O, Boon D, Lessler J. Variation in false-negative rate of reverse transcriptase polymerase chain reaction-based SARS-CoV-2 tests by time since exposure. *Ann Intern Med.* 2020;173(4):262-267.

10. Clark C. Fear of the false negative COVID-19 test. *Medpage Today.* 2020.

11. Hamblin J. Why COVID-19 makes some people so much sicker than others. *The Atlantic.* Published April 21, 2020.

12. Landon E. COVID-19: What we know so far about the 2019 novel coronavirus. *University of Chicago Medicine.* 2020.

13. World Health Organization. Report of the WHO-China Joint Mission on Coronavirus Disease 2019 (COVID-19). https://www.who.int/publications/i/item/report-of-the-who-china-joint-mission-on-coronavirus-disease-2019-(covid-19). Published February 28, 2020.

14. Chang, Mo G, Yuan X, et al. Time kinetics of viral clearance and resolution of symptoms in novel Coronavirus infection. *Am J Respir Crit Care Med.* 2020;201(9):1150-1152.

15. Lippi G, Sanchis-Gomar F, Henry BM. COVID-19: unravelling the clinical progression of nature's virtually perfect biological weapon. *Ann Transl Med.* 2020;8(11):693.

16. Coltrain N. Fact check: Does COVID-19 have a mortality rate of 1%-2%? *USA Today.* 2020.

17. Hannah Ritchie EO-O, Diana Beltekian, Edouard Mathieu, Joe Hasell, Bobbie Macdonald, Charlie Giattino, and Max Roser. Mortality risk of COVID-19. *Our World in Data.* 2020.

18. Centers for Disease Control and Prevention. Quarantine and isolation. https://www.cdc.gov/quarantine/index.html. Accessed 2020.

19. World Health Organization. "Immunity passports" in the context of COVID-19. https://www.who.int/news-room/commentaries/detail/immunity-passports-in-the-context-of-covid-19. Published April 24, 2020.

20. D'Ambrosio A. COVID-19 sequelae can linger for weeks. *MedPage Today*. Published May 13, 2020.

21. Zaim S, Chong JH, Sankaranarayanan V, Harky A. COVID-19 and multiorgan response. *Curr Probl Cardiol*. 2020;45(8):100618.

22. Wu Y, Xu X, Chen Z, et al. Nervous system involvement after infection with COVID-19 and other coronaviruses. *Brain Behav Immun*. 2020; 87:18-22.

23. Dubey S, Biswas P, Ghosh R, et al. Psychosocial impact of COVID-19. *Diabetes Metab Syndr*. 2020;14(5):779-788.

24. Centers for Disease Control and Prevention. Using Antibody Tests for COVID-19. https://www.cdc.gov/coronavirus/2019-ncov/lab/resources/antibody-tests.html. Updated May 28, 2020.

25. Marshall WF. How do COVID-19 antibody tests differ from diagnostic tests? *Mayo Clinic*. https://www.mayoclinic.org/covid-antibody-tests/expert-answers/faq-20484429. Published 2020.

26. Galiatsatos P. What coronavirus does to the lungs. Johns Hopkins Medicine. https://www.hopkinsmedicine.org/health/conditions-and-diseases/coronavirus/what-coronavirus-does-to-the-lungs. Published April 13, 2020. Accessed 2020.

27. AdventHealth. COVID-19: What are the long-term risks to your health? *AdventHealth*. https://www.adventhealth.com/blog/covid-19-what-are-long-term-risks-your-health. Published May 4, 2020.

28. Pesheva E. Coronavirus and the heart. https://hms.harvard.edu/news/coronavirus-heart.

Harvard Medical School. Published April 13, 2020. Accessed 2020.

29. Centers for Disease Control and Prevention. Coronavirus Disease 2019 (COVID-19): Frequently asked questions. https://www.cdc.gov/coronavirus/2019-ncov/faq.html. Published 2020.

AVAILABLE TREATMENTS

Is there a cure?

The simple answer is no. Currently, there are no Food and Drug Administration (FDA)-approved drugs for COVID-19.[1] With that said, there is an array of medications approved for other indications, as well as multiple investigational agents being studied for the treatment of SARS-CoV-2. In the case of the novel SARS-CoV-2 virus, the evidence to support medication use—which typically takes years to develop—is happening in real time parallel to the pandemic itself. In this setting, there has been much trial and error in formulating therapies that help fight this virus. The Centers for Disease Control (CDC) frequently updates its guidelines on recommended treatment based on well-designed clinical trials.[1] However, its recommendations are not considered mandates, and the choice of treatment for an individual patient should be decided by the patient with their doctor in the context of their unique circumstance.[1] There are several drugs currently being studied that have shown some benefit, particularly in the setting of severe or critical illness. However, the predominant therapy in regard to COVID-19 is based on supportive care for the patient.

What is the difference between treatment and cure?

A treatment is intended to reduce the severity or duration of a disease, which may reduce subsequent complications and morbidity. For example, HIV can be treated and managed but not cured. A cure eliminates disease. Many bacterial infections—for example, strep throat and chlamydia—are curable with antibiotics.

Currently, there are some treatments available for patients with COVID-19, but there is no cure.

What kind of care do patients with COVID-19 need?

The care needed is predominantly based on the illness severity. Patients infected with SARS-CoV-2 can be asymptomatic, meaning they test positive for the virus but show no symptoms. Patients who do develop symptoms can be clinically classified into mild, moderate, severe, or critical illness.[1] Although SARS-CoV-2 is considered primarily a respiratory virus, meaning it affects the lungs, the disease has the capability of generating a widespread inflammatory response impacting many organ systems in the body.

People who test positive for SARS-CoV-2 but are asymptomatic should self-isolate. If they remain asymptomatic, they can discontinue isolation seven days after the date of their positive test. If they become symptomatic, they should contact their physician for further guidance. No specific treatment is needed for asymptomatic patients.[1]

Patients with mild disease demonstrate symptoms such as fever, cough, sore throat, muscle aches, or headaches. However, they are typically without shortness of breath. If x-ray or CT images are obtained, the lungs may appear normal. Management in this case is non-specific and will involve treating symptoms. Patients with underlying medical problems—particularly those that affect their heart, lungs, liver, or kidneys—should be monitored closely for progression to a more severe disease process.[1]

Moderate illness is described as a progression to shortness of breath in combination with evidence of lung abnormalities on x-ray or CT scans. The threshold for hospitalization is lower in these cases because the likelihood of progression to severe disease is high. If there is suspicion for overlying bacterial pneumonia, antibiotics should be administered to the patient. Keeping the patient hydrated and monitoring their respiratory status is crucial.[1]

Severe illness is defined by increased shortness of breath, which can occur both with exertion and at rest. In-person evaluation is required and will often show oxygen saturation <93%, a breathing rate of >30 breaths/minute, and abnormal lung findings on x-ray or CT scan. These patients will require antibiotics if there is suspicion of a bacterial pneumonia superimposed on COVID-19. Additionally, giving the patient supplemental oxygen is typically required in patients with severe disease.[1]

Lastly, critically ill patients are those who experience life-threatening disease. This represents a widespread inflammatory process that promotes dysfunction not just in the lungs, but also in the heart, liver, kidneys, and brain. This has been discussed in the news as a "cytokine storm." When the body releases cytokines, or biochemical mediators that allow for communication between cells, they are essential in signaling the immune system to start doing its job. However, when this pathway is engaged too much, the immune system starts to damage the patient's normal tissue. The clinical hallmarks of cytokine storm are persistent fever and non-specific constitutional symptoms such as weight loss, muscle pain, fatigue, and headache. Progressive inflammation in this pathway leads to drops in blood pressure and progressive organ failure.[2] Unfortunately, there is no specific blood test to identify patients undergoing this phenomenon, but there are certain tests that can provide clues that a hyperactive inflammatory response is occurring. Management of these patients requires admitting the patient to a critical care unit for frequent monitoring of all their vital organs. Antibiotics, fluids, and oxygen will likely be administered, and the patient may require a ventilator that breathes for them.[1]

There are insufficient data to recommend either for or against any antiviral or immune modulating therapies in patients with COVID-19.[1]

Do we have any drugs that are effective against coronavirus?

There are currently no approved COVID-19 treatments. However, one drug that has received a lot of attention is the antiviral drug remdesivir. The coronavirus that causes COVID-19 is similar to the viruses that cause the diseases SARS (Severe Acute Respiratory Syndrome) and MERS (Middle East Respiratory Syndrome). Evidence from laboratory and animal studies suggests that remdesivir may help limit the reproduction and spread of these viruses in the body,[3] and a study published in the *New England Journal of Medicine* in May 2020 had promising results. In the study, over 1,000 people hospitalized with COVID-19 were randomized to receive either remdesivir or a placebo. Patients who received remdesivir recovered more rapidly than those who received the placebo, and this difference in recovery time was statistically significant.[3] Remdesivir seemed less effective in sicker patients, and it is unclear if the drug reduces mortality from COVID-19. In early May, the FDA approved emergency use authorization for remdesivir for adults and children hospitalized with severe COVID-19.[3] The CDC now recommends the use of remdesivir to treat COVID-19 in patients who require supplemental oxygen but are not mechanically ventilated (intubated).

A recent addition to the guidelines now recommends the use of dexamethasone, a corticosteroid, in patients who require supplemental oxygen but are not mechanically ventilated.

Convalescent plasma (the liquid component of blood) has been widely discussed as a potential treatment for COVID-19. Individuals who have been infected with SARS-CoV-2 will produce antibodies against the virus. Plasma from these individuals contains those antibodies. The thought is to use plasma from donors who have recovered from COVID-19 to help other sick patients suppress the virus and improve their immune response against it. However, there is still insufficient data to support the use of convalescent plasma.[1]

Several other drugs, including hydroxychloroquine, azithromycin, and other antiviral agents have been under study to determine their efficacy against COVID-19. Although there are some promising results, no drug is currently FDA-approved to treat COVID-19.[3]

Are hydroxychloroquine and azithromycin effective at preventing or treating COVID-19?

Early reports from China and France suggested that severe symptoms of COVID-19 improved more quickly when patients were given hydroxychloroquine. Some physicians gave a combination of hydroxychloroquine and azithromycin with some positive effects.[1]

Hydroxychloroquine is used primarily to treat malaria and several inflammatory autoimmune diseases, such as lupus and rheumatoid arthritis. Hydroxychloroquine can slow SARS-CoV-2 replication in laboratory studies[2]. It appears to work by two mechanisms: first, the drug makes it harder for the virus to attach to cells, which prevents it from entering cells and multiplying within them. Second, if the virus gets inside a cell, the drug prevents it from rapidly multiplying.[3]

Azithromycin is an antibiotic commonly prescribed for strep throat and bacterial pneumonia. It is not used for viral infections. However, it does have general anti-inflammatory properties. It has been proposed that azithromycin might slow the overactive inflammatory response seen in patients with COVID-19.[3]

There is not enough evidence yet on whether these drugs, alone or in combination, are effective at treating COVID-19. Although efficacious in the lab, these drugs have shown no benefit in humans.[2] *In vitro* studies, or those performed in laboratories, do not always translate to *in vivo* success, or the same results when used in the general public.

Regarding hydroxychloroquine specifically in preventing COVID-19, a recent *New England Journal of Medicine* clinical trial found that it did not prevent infection. However, this study has been questioned by some scientific experts.[3]

Where does this ultimately leave us? The recommendation outlined is that hydroxychloroquine and azithromycin, used either alone or in combination, should not be used to prevent or treat COVID-19 unless they are being prescribed in the hospital or as part of a clinical trial.[3]

Why do drugs need to be tested?

The Food and Drug Administration (FDA) Center for Drug Evaluation and Research (CEDER) evaluates drugs intended for human use to ensure that drugs marketed in the United States are safe and effective.[4] This process is also crucial for evaluating potential adverse reactions and side effects.

What steps are involved in drug testing?

Drug testing is typically a long process that takes years to accomplish. The process can be divided into pre-clinical and clinical phases. The pre-clinical phase predominantly involves simply discovering the drug and initial research and testing on non-human subjects. This process often takes three to six years.

Once the drug is approved for human testing, the clinical phase requires a four-step process, although FDA approval is granted after the third step.

- Step 1 involves a small number (20 to 80) of healthy volunteers or patients with the disease of interest. This goal of this step is to ask the simple question, *is the drug safe* for humans? This step assesses the drug's safety, as well as toxicities and understanding how the drug is metabolized by the body.

- Step 2 involves a larger number of participants, typically 100 to 300. This step primarily asks, *does the drug work?* In this part of testing, researchers will assess the efficacy, the best doses, and true adverse effects of the drug.
- Step 3 involves the largest number of participants (1,000 to 3,000), randomly assigned either to the drug under investigation or to the current treatment or placebo. Step 3 confirms safety and effectiveness of the drug. After step 3, the drug undergoes FDA review for approval.
- Step 4 occurs after FDA approval when the drug is out on the market. This part of testing looks at whether the drug will stay or be withdrawn from the marketplace. Also, as time goes on, rare or long-term (blackbox) effects may be discovered.[5]

In some cases, approval of a new drug is expedited. This is applied to promising therapies that can treat a serious or life-threatening condition. This is a pathway for a COVID-19 vaccine which is imperative to providing immunity to the population at large and greatly slowing the spread of the virus.[6]

What is a randomized controlled trial?

A randomized controlled trial is a research study in which people are allocated at random (by chance) to receive one of several clinical interventions; for example, a new medication to treat high blood pressure versus a placebo. The experimental group receives a drug of interest and the other group, the control, receives a placebo where no true intervention is occurring at all or, sometimes, a different active treatment. Randomized controlled trials are also typically blinded, meaning that participants are not aware of which group they belong to. Randomized controlled trials seek to compare the outcomes after the participants receive the intervention. The use of randomization to determine which patients are in which group is a powerful way to prevent bias from affecting the study results. Randomized controlled trials are one of the simplest and most powerful tools in clinical research.[7]

Are antibiotics effective?

SARS-CoV-2 is a virus and will not directly respond to antibiotics. However, when a virus attacks someone's lungs, this often creates an environment susceptible to bacterial pneumonia. If this is the case, patients will benefit from antibiotic therapy to help treat the specific bacterial component of their illness. With that said, there is still no evidence that supports the use of antibiotics in COVID-19.

What is the likelihood of needing a ventilator?

This is a difficult question to answer. Initial studies on COVID-19 suggest that the overall likelihood of needing a ventilator is relatively low. Like many other disease processes, a patient's baseline health profile plays a large role in how likely they are to develop severe sequelae of COVID-19. The majority of patients who contract the virus will not require hospital admission because they will either be asymptomatic or only experience mild disease. Those with moderate or severe disease processes will likely require hospital admission. However, only a small percentage of patients in the hospital will need intensive care, which often means being put on a ventilator. Initial reports suggest that about 5% of proven COVID-19 positive patients will require intensive care.

However, there have only been a handful of studies detailing the percentage of patients requiring ventilation. The first detailed study of COVID-19 patients in China showed only a 2.3% chance of requiring ventilation. A subsequent study in New York City found that 12.2% of patients required mechanical ventilation.[8] Patients who are likely to require advanced care tend to be older and have comorbid conditions—commonly diabetes, cardiac disease, or underlying lung problems.

Rates of hospital admission, requirement of intensive care, or ventilation are difficult to truly quantify because testing is still limited, and case rates across geographic regions are so variable. Preliminary data suggest that the majority of patients do not require hospital admission and can be managed conservatively at home. Of patients with more severe disease that need to be managed in the hospital, less than half need intensive care or mechanical ventilation.

References

1. COVID-19 Treatment Guidelines Panel. Coronavirus disease 2019 (COVID-19) treatment guidelines. National Institutes of Health. Available at https://www.covid19treatmentguidelines.nih.gov/. Accessed June 9, 2020

2. Mangalmurti N, Hunter C. Cytokine storms: Understanding COVID-19. *Immunity, 53*(1), 19-25.

3. Harvard Health Publishing. Treatments for COVID-19. https://www.health.harvard.edu/diseases-and-conditions/treatments-for-covid-19. Accessed June 8, 2020.

4. Center for Drug Evaluation and Research. Frequently asked questions about the FDA drug approval process. https://www.fda.gov/drugs/special-features/frequently-asked-questions-about-fda-drug-approval-process. Accessed June 8, 2020.

5. Le T, Bhushan V, Sochat M. First aid for the USMLE step 1 2019. New York: McGraw-Hill Education.

6. Center for Drug Evaluation and Research. Drug development & approval process. https://www.fda.gov/drugs/development-approval-process-drugs. Accessed June 10, 2020.

7. Shiel, W. Definition of randomized controlled trial. https://www.medicinenet.com/script/main/art.asp?articlekey=39532. Accessed June 14, 2020.

8. Richardson S, Hirsch JS, Narasimhan M, et al. Presenting characteristics, comorbidities, and outcomes among 5700 patients hospitalized with COVID-19 in the New York City area. *JAMA*. 2020;323(20):2052–2059.

VACCINES

How do vaccines work?

Before discussing vaccines, it is important to understand some basic functions of the immune system. The immune system defends the body from disease-causing pathogens, and it accomplishes this through two separate divisions: innate immunity and adaptive immunity. Innate immunity is automatic and has no memory, meaning it will respond immediately and without discrimination against foreign substances. Adaptive immunity is slower and does have memory, meaning that it takes time to mount a response against a foreign invader, and the body will "recognize" the invader if it is encountered again. Because the adaptive immune system recognizes the invader on subsequent encounters, it can quickly neutralize or eliminate the threat.

Vaccines work by training the adaptive immune system to recognize and fight off pathogens, which are typically either viruses or bacteria.[1] Essentially, vaccination promotes immunity by imitating an infection.[2] Vaccines are often made with very small amounts of weakened or killed germ—which, if at full strength, would have the potential to cause disease—or with small parts of the virus that are not at all capable of causing infection. Through vaccination, the body recognizes these as foreign invaders and responds by producing immune cells and antibodies that kill the germs. It typically takes several days for the body to mount an immune response after vaccination. Therefore, if you contract a virus just before or just after vaccination against said virus, you may develop the full-blown disease because the vaccine has not had enough time to provide protection.[2]

One of the most important benefits of vaccination is that it stimulates the production of memory cells, which "remember" how to fight the disease that was vaccinated against if it is encountered in the future. This means if you are exposed to the real virus or bacteria after vaccination, your body will be able to recognize and attack these pathogens more quickly and aggressively than if you were not vaccinated, preventing the virus or bacteria from causing serious disease.[1]

What is the difference between a live attenuated vaccine and an inactivated vaccine?

A live attenuated vaccine uses a weakened, but still living, form of a virus or bacterium that causes disease. The term "attenuated" means that the pathogen's ability to cause an infection has been reduced.[3] Because this form of vaccine is the closest thing to a natural infection, it can create a strong and long-lasting immune response.[4] However, live attenuated vaccines need extensive safety testing.[3] Some live attenuated viruses can revert back to their original forms or to a form that is capable of causing disease via mutations.[5] Therefore, people who have weakened immune systems—for example, people with long-term health problems or people who have had an organ transplant—should consult their physician before receiving this type of vaccination, and some people will not be able to receive these vaccines at all.[4]

An inactivated vaccine uses a killed version of the germ that causes a disease. The injectable flu vaccine is an example of an inactivated vaccine. This type of vaccine can trigger an immune response, but it cannot cause an infection.[3] The killed (or inactive) pathogens cannot revert to a more virulent form that is capable of causing disease.[5] Therefore, this type of vaccine can be safely given to people who have impaired immune systems. However, inactivated vaccines usually provide shorter and weaker protection compared with live attenuated vaccines. Hence, multiple doses of vaccine followed by occasional booster doses are often needed to provide lasting immunity.[3]

There are many other types of vaccines—including RNA, DNA, and protein subunit vaccines—but most common and well-known vaccines are either inactivated or live attenuated.[6]

Can a vaccine cause COVID-19?

It is very unlikely that a vaccine will be able to cause COVID-19; vaccines are extremely safe and effective because they are extensively tested. Since they are administered to enormous portions of the population and are typically given to healthy people, even a very small chance of causing harm would affect many people and undermine the public's trust in vaccination. For these reasons, vaccines undergo rigorous safety testing before they are approved by the FDA. A vaccine for COVID-19 would be held to the same standards despite the pressure of a global pandemic. In fact, the immense pressure of developing a COVID-19 vaccine has led to intense scrutiny of safety practices, as any misstep might jeopardize public trust and result in fewer people receiving the vaccine.

The chance that a vaccine can cause disease is extremely low, as many vaccines are inactivated (or killed) vaccines that are incapable of causing disease. Live attenuated vaccines—which contain weakened forms of germs—typically do not cause disease in healthy people, although occasionally children can develop a very mild rash and fever following vaccination with the MMR, MMRV, or varicella vaccines.[7] All of these vaccines undergo testing to ensure that the virus used in the vaccine is not capable of causing disease.[8]

The benefits of vaccines vastly outweigh their risks. The risk of serious harm from vaccines is orders of magnitude lower than the risks posed by the diseases they protect against.[9] For example, vaccination against diphtheria with the DTaP vaccine causes severe fever (greater than 105°F) in approximately 1 in 16,000 children.[10] However, diphtheria itself will kill 1-2 people for every 20 with the disease.[10] In young children, the case-fatality rate is even higher—up to 1 in 5. Public vaccination programs have all but eradicated many infectious diseases which, without vaccination, have great potential to cause lifelong disability or death.[10]

What is herd immunity and why is it important?

Herd immunity means that once enough people in a community are immune to an infectious disease, either through vaccination or natural infection, opportunities for spreading the disease from person to person become very low. When herd immunity is achieved, the average number of new infections caused by an infectious person, or R_0, will be less than 1. This will cause daily new cases to decline.[11] When a virus does not have enough susceptible hosts to establish a foothold, it eventually dies out completely.[1] This is how herd immunity helps reduce viral transmission and can control a pandemic.

Establishing herd immunity is one of the most effective ways to prevent outbreaks of infectious diseases such as measles, mumps, polio, and chickenpox. More importantly, herd immunity helps provide indirect protection to people who cannot get vaccinated and are vulnerable to disease such as babies, pregnant women, and people who are immunocompromised.[12]

Is herd immunity possible? What would it take to achieve herd immunity from SARS-CoV-2?

In order to achieve herd immunity, the majority of the population either needs to receive a protective vaccine or recover from infection. Based on a study from Los Alamos National Laboratory, the R_0 for SARS-CoV-2 may be as high as 5.7, which would mean that at least 82% of the population needs to be immune to reach herd protection.[13,14]

There are several ways to achieve herd immunity:

- **Worst case scenario:** we do not perform social distancing or enact other measures to slow down the spread of COVID-19. The virus infects as many people as possible within a few months, growing exponentially, which overwhelms hospitals and leads to high death rates. Those who survive the infection presumably achieve immunity.

- **Best case scenario:** we maintain or reduce current viral transmission rates through a concerted effort by the entire population. This requires wearing masks, following public health guidelines, and maintaining social distancing for an extended period of time until a highly effective vaccine becomes available and most of the population receives it.
- **Most likely scenario:** we perform some social distancing, and infection rates rise and fall over time. This would require easing or tightening social distancing measures depending on the circumstances. Prolonged efforts would be required to prevent outbreaks until an effective vaccine is developed, tested, and mass produced. Herd immunity would result from a mixture of vaccination and natural infection.[15]

Is a vaccine possible?

Yes, several vaccines to prevent SARS-CoV-2 infection are hurtling through development at record speed.[16] In early July 2020, more than 140 vaccines were under development from government scientists, biotech companies, and university researchers.[17] Thirteen of these vaccines were being tested in human clinical trials.[18] Some vaccine developers, including a research group in China and the U.S. biotech company Moderna, have already posted preliminary but promising results from their vaccine trials.[19]

As of late July 2020, Moderna has started phase 3 clinical trials for its vaccine candidate. 30,000 trial participants will be recruited to test for vaccine efficacy and potential adverse effects. Moderna hopes to complete this trial in October 2020 and is producing millions of doses of vaccine in parallel, with the intent of immediately distributing the vaccine if trial results are promising.

How long will it take to develop a vaccine?

Typically, the process of vaccine development takes at least 10 years. The fastest modern vaccine ever developed was the Ebola vaccine, which took four years. The fact that a COVID-19 vaccine has already progressed to human clinical trials in less than a year is an incredible feat, and this is by far the fastest a vaccine has ever been developed.[17]

Dr. Anthony Fauci, the U.S. government's leading vaccine expert and director of the National Institute of Allergy and Infectious Diseases, is optimistic that a COVID-19 vaccine will be widely available by early 2021.[20]

Why does vaccine development take so long?

A potential COVID-19 vaccine needs to undergo extensive safety testing before being administered to millions, if not billions, of people. The goals are to ensure that the vaccine is safe, provides long-term protection, and adequately protects elderly people, who are at high risk from COVID-19 and tend to respond less robustly to vaccination.[3]

Developing a vaccine that is both effective and safe is grueling and methodical work. Vaccine candidates must first be tested in animals and then in humans in three different phases. Human clinical trials are composed of three phases. During a phase 1 clinical trial, the vaccine is given to a small group of people to test whether the vaccine is safe. During a phase 2 clinical trial, a larger number of people receive the vaccine to see if it works and to determine possible side effects. Vaccines that progress to phase 3 clinical trials are given to an even larger group of people, typically in an outbreak area, where vaccine efficacy and potential adverse effects are monitored.[21] Vaccines that pass phase 3 clinical trials are approved by the FDA, and then it takes time to produce, distribute, and administer the vaccine to the global population.[3]

If vaccine development is usually so slow, how are COVID-19 vaccines developing so rapidly?

Despite the lengthy process of vaccine development, there is a global effort underway to accelerate development due to the seriousness of the COVID-19 pandemic. Governments and regulatory bodies are shortening the timeline by prioritizing the review of COVID-19-related data, dedicating committees to application review, combining classical phase 1 and phase 2 clinical trials into a single trial protocol, and running trials in parallel rather than sequentially.[22] These steps help save valuable time in early clinical development by reducing administrative burden and lengthy review processes, enabling researchers to rapidly move forward to pivotal trials if the vaccine candidate appears to be safe and effective.[22] Many researchers are optimistic that a COVID-19 vaccine will arrive faster than ever before in vaccine history.[19]

If a vaccine is possible, will it be effective?

It is likely the vaccine will be effective, but it is impossible to say *how* effective it will be.[3] In the best case scenario, the vaccine response will produce enough neutralizing antibodies to prevent viral infection entirely, providing what is called "sterilizing immunity."[23] In less optimal scenarios, people who receive the vaccine may still experience mild disease when exposed to the virus, or they may be able to infect others while sick. For example, the flu vaccine often cannot protect entirely against the flu, but it can reduce the severity of disease. Getting a flu shot remains one of the best possible ways to prevent severe influenza despite the shot's inability to provide sterilizing immunity.[24]

Early vaccine trials have shown promising results, and several vaccine candidates have successfully produced an antibody response against SARS-CoV-2.[25] Even if a COVID-19 vaccine ultimately cannot prevent infection, these antibodies will likely reduce disease severity and complications if infection occurs.

Would a vaccine have to be given yearly, like the flu vaccine?

It is not clear if a COVID-19 vaccine would need to be given yearly, as none have received FDA approval yet. Flu vaccination is needed yearly because flu viruses are constantly changing; therefore, the vaccine must be updated annually to protect against the strains of influenza that scientists anticipate will be the most common during an upcoming flu season.[26]

Given the number of COVID-19 vaccine trials underway, it is likely that more than one vaccine will eventually obtain FDA approval. Therefore, the amount of protection each vaccine provides may vary.[19] Fortunately, SARS-CoV-2 does not mutate as rapidly as the influenza virus, which makes it unlikely that a vaccine against COVID-19 would need to be administered annually.[8,27]

If a vaccine is developed, who would get it first?

Multiple public health organizations have established frameworks for vaccine distribution during a pandemic. As vaccines initially become available, they may be a scarce resource, and vaccination priority will be determined with the goal of reducing mortality and protecting healthcare systems.[28]

The World Health Organization (WHO) has proposed a tiered system of COVID-19 vaccination that prioritizes healthcare workers, then adults over the age of 65, and then adults with high risk comorbidities before proceeding to vaccination of the general public. Geography and population vulnerability will also be factors in determining initial allocation of resources.[28]

The Centers for Disease Control (CDC) has not produced a framework specific to COVID-19 but may adapt existing prioritization guidelines that were originally produced for pandemic influenza. The CDC guidelines are more complicated than the WHO guidelines and take into account occupational group as well as risk level. Under the CDC guidelines, top priority is given to healthcare workers, deployed military personnel, emergency services and law enforcement officers, pregnant women, infants, and toddlers.[29]

In both cases, essential healthcare workers are prioritized and will likely be among the first groups to be vaccinated. However, final decisions regarding who will get the vaccine first will vary among states, and the CDC will need to collaborate with local health departments to ensure that vaccine allocation adequately covers target groups and at-risk communities.[29,30]

If a vaccine is developed, what would we know about it? What would we not know?

If and when a vaccine is developed, we will be one step closer to achieving herd immunity, which will help reduce the risk of contracting COVID-19 and the risk of experiencing severe symptoms if infection occurs.[31]

However, we do not know if this immunity will protect against repeated viral infection. Due to SARS-CoV-2's potential for mutation, antibodies that are effective against one strain of the virus may not work against variants that develop in the future.[32] In addition, we do not know how long any immunity might last. We may need to give booster shots to produce long-lasting immunity.[33]

Finally, completing vaccine trials may prove to be the easy part of the process. Long-term safety data would be desirable but will likely not be available when mass vaccination campaigns begin. A robust public health campaign rooted in the safety of and trust in a COVID-19 vaccine may be needed to get enough people vaccinated to provide an adequate level of herd immunity.

I heard about a Russian vaccine receiving approval. What are some details about that vaccine?

On August 11, 2020, Russia's Ministry of Health approved a COVID-19 vaccine nicknamed "Sputnik V," a reference to the world's first artificial satellite launched by the Soviet Union during the Cold War.[34] Despite Russia's claims of safety and efficacy, the vaccine has not completed clinical trials and had only been tested in 76 people at the time of approval.[34] The approval has been widely condemned by the scientific community as premature and lacking in safety data.

According to the Gamaleya Institute—the Russian institute that developed the vaccine—20 countries had placed orders for over 1 billion doses of the vaccine within a day of the vaccine's approval.[35] Within Russia, the vaccine can be administered immediately to vulnerable groups (e.g., the elderly and medical workers) but widespread vaccination campaigns will not begin until January 2021.[34] This will presumably allow for the completion of a phase 3 clinical trial which began on August 12.[34] It is unlikely that Western democracies and other developed countries will adopt the vaccine without extensive safety testing and completion of clinical trials.

References

1. How vaccines work. PublicHealth.org. https://www.publichealth.org/public-awareness/understanding-vaccines/vaccines-work/. Published 2020. Accessed June 9, 2020.

2. Centers for Disease Control and Prevention. Understanding how vaccines work. https://www.cdc.gov/vaccines/hcp/conversations/understanding-vacc-work.html. Published August 17, 2018. Accessed June 9, 2020.

3. Mayo Clinic. COVID-19 (Coronavirus) Vaccine: Get the Facts. https://www.mayoclinic.org/diseases-conditions/coronavirus/in-depth/coronavirus-vaccine/art-20484859. Published May 8, 2020. Accessed June 9, 2020.

4. U.S. Department of Health and Human Services. Vaccine types. https://www.vaccines.gov/basics/types. Published March 2020. Accessed June 16, 2020.

5. Different Types of Vaccines. History of Vaccines. https://www.historyofvaccines.org/content/articles/ different-types-vaccines. Published January 17, 2018. Accessed June 16, 2020.

6. Palca J. All you wanted to know about coronavirus vaccine science but were afraid to ask. NPR. https://www.npr.org/sections/health-shots/2020/06/ 24/881704736/all-you-wanted-to-know-about-coron- avirus-vaccine-science-but-were-afraid-to-ask. Pub- lished June 24, 2020. Accessed July 22, 2020.

7. Vaccines: Common concerns. Caring for kids. https://www.caringforkids.cps.ca/handouts/vaccines- common-concerns. Published November 2016. Ac- cessed June 16, 2020.

8. Nania R. Coronavirus Vaccine: When will we have one, who gets it and will it work? AARP. https://www.aarp.org/health/conditions-treatments/ info-2020/coronavirus-vaccine-research.html. Pub- lished June 5, 2020. Accessed June 9, 2020.

9. Centers for Disease Control and Prevention. U.S. Vac- cine Safety - Overview, history, and how it works. https://www.cdc.gov/vaccinesafety/ensuringsafety/ history/index.html. Published July 1, 2020. Accessed July 22, 2020.

10. Diphtheria. Vaccines. https://www.vaccines.gov/dis- eases/diphtheria. Accessed July 28, 2020.

11. Science Media Centre. Expert comments about herd immunity. https://www.sciencemediacentre.org/ex- pert-comments-about-herd-immunity/. Published March 13, 2020. Accessed June 16, 2020.

12. Association for Professionals in Infection Control and Epidemiology. Herd immunity. https://apic.org/monthly_alerts/herd-immunity/. Published August 25, 2015. Accessed June 9, 2020.

13. Sanche S, Lin Y, Xu C, et al. High Contagiousness and Rapid Spread of Severe Acute Respiratory Syndrome Coronavirus 2. *Emerging Infectious Diseases.* 2020;26(7):1470-1477.

14. Biggers A, Ramirez VB. What Is R0? Gauging contagious infections. Healthline. https://www.healthline.com/health/r-nought-reproduction-number. Published April 20, 2020. Accessed June 16, 2020.

15. D'Souza G, Dowdy D. What is herd immunity and how can we achieve it with COVID-19? Johns Hopkins Bloomberg School of Public Health. https://www.jhsph.edu/covid-19/articles/achieving-herd-immunity-with-covid19.html. Published April 10, 2020. Accessed June 9, 2020.

16. Branswell H. Mounting promises on Covid-19 vaccines are fueling false expectations, experts say. *STAT.* https://www.statnews.com/2020/05/06/mounting-promises-on-covid-vaccines/. Published May 6, 2020. Accessed June 9, 2020.

17. Farris M. COVID-19 Vaccine possible by early 2021, Local Expert Says. *4WWL.* https://www.wwltv.com/article/news/health/coronavirus/covid-19-vaccine-possible-by-early-2021-local-expert-sayd/289-1638e3da-3a64-4442-a15b-9abceb248e2f. Published May 20, 2020. Accessed June 9, 2020.

18. Campbell M. 13 COVID-19 vaccines are in human clinical trials – What are they? Biopharma from Technology Networks. https://www.technologynetworks.com/biopharma/blog/13-covid-19-vaccines-are-in-human-clinical-trials-what-are-they-336738. Published June 29, 2020. Accessed July 22, 2020.

19. Irfan U. Why a vaccine may not be enough to end the pandemic. Vox. https://www.vox.com/2020/6/3/21258841/coronavirus-vaccine-covid-19-testing-usa-china-moderna. Published June 3, 2020. Accessed June 9, 2020.

20. Booker B. Fauci says it's 'doable' to have millions of doses of COVID-19 vaccine by January. NPR. https://www.npr.org/sections/coronavirus-live-updates/2020/04/30/848478507/fauci-says-its-doable-to-have-millions-of-doses-of-covid-19-vaccine-by-january. Published April 30, 2020. Accessed June 9, 2020.

21. Simon M. Why creating a Covid-19 vaccine is taking so long. Wired. https://www.wired.com/story/why-creating-a-covid-19-vaccine-is-taking-so-long/. Published May 20, 2020. Accessed June 9, 2020.

22. van der Plas JL, Roestenberg M, Cohen AF, Kamerling IMC. How to expedite early-phase SARS-CoV-2 vaccine trials in pandemic setting-A practical perspective [published online ahead of print, 2020 Jun 19]. Br J Clin Pharmacol. 2020;10.1111/bcp.14435.

23. Hou C-Y. What is sterilizing immunity and do we need it for the coronavirus? *TheHill.* https://thehill.com/changing-america/well-being/prevention-

cures/501677-what-is-sterilizing-immunity-and-do-we-need-it. Published June 8, 2020. Accessed July 22, 2020.

24. Roche GC. Flu vaccine reduces virus severity in patients, regardless of prevention. HCP Live. https://www.mdmag.com/medical-news/flu-vaccine-reduces-virus-severity-patients-prevention. Published January 23, 2019. Accessed July 22, 2020.

25. Etherington D. COVID-19 vaccine trials from the University of Oxford and Wuhan both show early positive results. TechCrunch. https://techcrunch.com/2020/07/20/covid-19-vaccine-trials-from-the-university-of-oxford-and-wuhan-both-show-early-positive-results/. Published July 20, 2020. Accessed July 22, 2020.

26. Centers for Disease Control and Prevention. Key facts abouts flu vaccine. https://www.cdc.gov/flu/prevent/keyfacts.htm. Published April 28, 2020. Accessed June 16, 2020.

27. Crist C. Annual COVID-19 vaccine may be necessary. WebMD. https://www.webmd.com/lung/news/20200504/--annual_covid-19-vaccine-may-be-necessary. Published May 4, 2020. Accessed June 9, 2020.

28. World Health Organization. A global framework to ensure equitable and fair allocation of COVID-19 products and potential implications for COVID-19 vaccines. Published June 18, 2020. Accessed July 22, 2020.

29. Centers for Disease Control and Prevention. Interim Updated Planning Guidance on Allocating and Targeting Pandemic Influenza Vaccine During an Influenza

Pandemic. 2018. https://www.cdc.gov/flu/pandemic-resources/pdf/2018-Influenza-Guidance.pdf.

30. Jauhar S. With a Covid-19 vaccine in hand, who should get it first? STAT. https://www.statnews.com/2020/05/23/when-a-covid-19-vaccine-becomes-avail-able-who-should-get-it-first/. Published May 23, 2020. Accessed June 9, 2020.

31. Branswell H. The world may be overestimating the power of Covid-19 vaccines. STAT. https://www.stat-news.com/2020/05/22/the-world-needs-covid-19-vac-cines-it-may-also-be-overestimating-their-power/. Published May 22, 2020. Accessed June 16, 2020.

32. Lai J. What we still don't know: Here are some of the big coronavirus questions scientists are racing to an-swer. *The Philadelphia Inquirer.* https://www.in-quirer.com/health/coronavirus/coronavirus-covid19-questions-research-immunity-treatment-vaccines-20200427.html. Published May 5, 2020. Accessed June 9, 2020.

33. Palca J. When can we expect a coronavirus vaccine? NPR. https://www.npr.org/sections/goatsandsoda/2020/05/12/852886535/when-can-we-expect-a-coro-navirus-vaccine. Published May 12, 2020. Accessed June 16, 2020.

34. Cohen J. Russia's approval of a COVID-19 vaccine is less than meets the press release. *Science.* https://www.sciencemag.org/news/2020/08/russia-s-approval-covid-19-vaccine-less-meets-press-release. Published Aug 11, 2020. Accessed Aug 13, 2020.

35. Kramer, A. Russia approves coronavirus vaccine before completing tests. *The New York Times.* https://www.nytimes.com/2020/08/11/world/europe/russia-coronavirus-vaccine-approval.html. Published Aug 11, 2020. Accessed Aug 13, 2020.

REOPENING

What are some arguments for reopening businesses?

The strongest argument for reopening businesses is to reduce the impact COVID-19 has had on the economy. At the national scale, it is easy to see the economic effects COVID-19 has produced. Since March 1, nearly 20% of the labor force in the US has filed for unemployment insurance, and the unemployment rate has reached a staggering 14.7% from 3.8% in February 2020.[1] This will continue to increase as small businesses are strained by public health restrictions. Small businesses are not the only ones suffering during COVID-19; many big-name companies are filing for bankruptcy as well, including Brooks Brothers, Gold's Gym, JCPenney, multiple airlines, and several oil companies.[2] Reopening businesses could potentially reduce the impact of COVID-19 on the economy.

On a smaller and more local scale, individuals and small businesses will likely feel the blow of COVID-19 the most. People who lose their jobs due to COVID-19 may not have enough money to pay for housing or feed their families. In addition, many people have lost their health insurance because health insurance is often employment-based. Unemployment has many negative indirect health consequences when people cannot afford to eat nutritious food, live in a safe environment, or see the doctor.

A Cowles Foundation discussion paper, produced by Yale University, surveyed over 8,000 small businesses and found that 60% had had to lay off at least one employee due to COVID-19. The same survey also found that 46% of small business owners feel that it will take at least two years to recover from the impact of COVID-19.[3] Allowing small businesses to reopen could help prevent them from failing and allow more people to continue working.

What are some arguments for reopening schools?

Along with the negative economic impacts of strict lockdowns, keeping schools closed limits many adults' ability to work because they must look after their children rather than sending them to schools and daycares. Providing childcare is a full-time job, which limits one or both parents' ability to participate in the official workforce.[4] In addition, SARS-CoV-2 appears to be less contagious among young children, and children who contract the virus are much less likely to have severe disease than adults.[5] According to the Centers for Disease Control and Prevention (CDC), as of July 2020, only 0.03% of the total COVID-19 deaths in the US were children under the age of 15.[6] This relatively low risk is why elementary and middle schools in France are reopening, while high schools are remaining closed and learning will be done online. The French government believes that in the long run, time off from school will be more detrimental for students than holding conventional classes.[7] (However, France has substantially less community spread and greater adherence to public health guidelines than the United States.)

Although online education is a realistic option for older students—those in high school and above—it is not without considerable challenges. Children in poorer households may not have access to the Internet and necessary technology, which makes online learning and homework less feasible. Virtual schooling also does not allow children to socialize with one another, which is an important contributor to the mental health of children and teens. Online classes may also be less effective: a survey done by Niche, a company that specializes in analyzing education from grade school through college, found that only 11% of high school students feel that online classes are as effective as in-person classes.[8] Many of these points may lead our country to open schools back up with precautions to limit the spread of COVID-19.

What are some arguments for keeping businesses and schools closed with limited services?

Reopening businesses and schools will increase the risk of exposure to the 5% of the population that is most susceptible to SARS-CoV-2. This is roughly 16.5 million people in the U.S. People who have chronic health problems—such as COPD, heart failure, and immunocompromising conditions, among many others—fall into this category. This population overwhelmed healthcare systems in New York City in March and April.[9]

Although individuals outside of this high-risk population are less susceptible to severe disease, they are still at risk. From February 1 to June 17, 20,064 individuals below the age of 65 died from COVID-19 in the U.S.[10] This represented 19.41% of all COVID-19 deaths in the U.S. at the time, meaning the virus is dangerous across age groups. Opening businesses and other facilities too quickly will cause an increase in cases, which will increase the number of deaths and potentially overburden healthcare systems.[10]

Opening schools without limitations also has its challenges. Although children are not at great risk of suffering from the virus, they will increase the spread of SARS-CoV-2 even if their ability to spread the virus is low. Eventually, if the virus continues to spread at a rapid rate, it will burden the economy. A large spike in COVID-19 cases may precipitate another shutdown, and even if a shutdown does not occur, people who do not feel safe in public are not likely to dine at restaurants, travel, or participate in activities that require contact with others. Ultimately, this surge would undermine all the public health measures and sacrifice of the first shutdown, postponing any meaningful economic and educational recovery. This is why public health experts propose a cautious, limited, and slow reopening.

What might the workplace look like post-COVID-19?

Dramatic world events often shape social norms and how we interact with the world. For example, WWII created a vacancy in the labor force that drove women into the workforce. Even after WWII ended, many women continued to work instead of returning to the previous norm. After 9/11, another society-changing event, national security increased dramatically and led to substantially increased airport security protocols and the creation of the Department of Homeland Security.

COVID-19 will probably bring many changes that will last long after the pandemic is over.

With many states issuing stay-at-home orders, businesses have had to adapt to employees working remotely. Remote work has demonstrated that for many workers, it is not necessary to work in an office five days a week. This could drive many businesses to continue working remotely post-COVID-19, particularly among tech companies and professions such as programming and web design. In areas where office space is expensive, increasing the amount of time employees work from home may be cost-effective for companies. We may also see staggering of employee schedules as more individuals work from home. People may work staggered hours or staggered days to accommodate a downsized office space. If these changes occur, they may lead to secondary impacts, such as decreased demand for office real estate, less traffic, and less need for public transportation in some areas.[11]

What might schools look like post-COVID-19?

As schools start to reopen, many precautions will be necessary. After COVID-19, we may see a shift to more virtual learning. Like anything, there are pros and cons to online learning. Some of the downsides to virtual learning are that the quality of online courses relies heavily on teacher's technological capabilities, it is more difficult for teachers to engage their students without a physical presence, students can easily access their phones and Internet during class, and it is difficult for teachers to manage student behavior during virtual classes. Online learning is also not compatible with every subject—classes like art, theater, and woodshop will either be severely affected or non-existent in an online curriculum.

These are just a few of the challenges associated with online learning. However, although there are many barriers to online learning, there are also many benefits.

One of the benefits of online learning is the potential integration of learning and multimedia. The more we integrate learning with different senses, the more we retain. Hearing a lecture alone is less effective than hearing a lecture while also seeing visuals that incorporate the information. Using technology to make learning more interactive can improve the quality of education. Online learning is also convenient: students do not have to leave their homes if all their needs are met there. Another benefit of virtual learning is that students who are typically shy may be more active in discussions when they can use the chat function on learning platforms. Distributing information and assignments would be easier for the teacher and the learners.[12] Based on these pros and cons, the utility of online learning will likely vary depending on the age and independence of the learner.

In higher education—generally, college and university—students are more independent and should need little direction when it comes to staying on task and prioritizing their schedules. In these settings, we may see a blend of online classes with in-person workshops. In a survey done by the company Niche, approval of online classes during COVID-19 among this age group was 72%, which was the highest approval rating out of all age groups.[13] The pandemic has also affected other aspects of higher education such as admissions exams. Before the pandemic, many undergraduate and graduate institutions were considering getting rid of standardized tests like the SAT, ACT, and MCAT as criteria for admission. This year, due to COVID-19-related testing center closures and general disruption, even more schools have made it optional to submit test scores with applications.[14] This may serve as a test run for many institutions, and it may lead to many more schools either getting rid of these tests entirely or making them optional for applicants.

In high school, we may see a mix of in-class and online learning. High school students are often independent enough that they can work from home without too much adult supervision. Generally, they are also resourceful and savvy enough with technology to properly utilize online tools. We might see in-class time used for classes that involve workshops or those that are more kinetic (e.g., woodshop, physical education, art). A select group of students may resume school in traditional classrooms—this could include students who have difficulty staying on task or students who are struggling with grades or behavior.

In contrast, children in eighth grade and under are far less independent, so a mixed curriculum is unlikely to be feasible. Young children need more assistance, supervision, and socialization, which is foundational in early years of development.[15] Most parents will still have to work, and an at-home virtual classroom would make this particularly challenging. At this point nothing is certain, but regardless of the pandemic's outcome, we will likely see changes to classroom structure and the incorporation of virtual learning.

What is meant by a phased reopening?

A phased reopening means letting businesses and society open incrementally as certain criteria are met. The decisions regarding reopening are dictated by individual states. When state governments have a grasp on how the virus is spreading in their state, they can focus on regional transmission patterns, moving cities and towns forward or backward in the reopening process based on epidemiologic metrics. For example, for a state to even begin the first phase of reopening, there must be a downward trend in new cases per day over 14 days, among other criteria. These criteria are in place to prevent another surge of the virus and reduce the risk of overburdening healthcare systems. Once the phases begin, it is still imperative to practice good hygiene, social distancing, and to self-isolate if you are feeling sick. If progressing to a new phase causes too great of a spike in cases, states will either halt reopening or move back to a previous phase. California, for example, had to tighten restrictions after COVID-19 cases surged in July.

The U.S. government has proposed a 3-phase system. In phase 1, vulnerable populations should continue to shelter in place if possible. This includes the elderly, transplant patients, cancer patients, and other immunocompromised individuals. Healthy individuals should still try to minimize exposure, but non-essential travel can resume. Businesses have their own set of guidelines during phase 1. Businesses should try to maintain telework whenever possible and make accommodations for social distancing if employees must physically go to work. Facilities that should remain closed include schools and daycares as well as large venues like movie theaters, gyms, and sit-down restaurants. Hospitals cannot permit visitors and should only perform elective surgeries if the hospital is capable of handling a surge of COVID-19 patients. Once the state meets epidemiological criteria, it may move on to phase 2.

Phase 2 is remarkably similar to phase 1. Immunocompromised individuals should continue to shelter in place. Facilities containing vulnerable populations such as hospitals and nursing homes should have strict visiting policies and infection control measures. Healthy individuals should continue to practice proper social distancing. Businesses such as daycares can reopen, and large venues can reopen as long as strict sanitation and social distancing measures are in place. Bars and restaurants can reopen with diminished capacity. Once further criteria are met, states can move on to phase 3.

In phase 3, vulnerable populations can go out in public, but are advised to do so with caution. Nursing homes and hospitals with strict hygiene measures in place can allow visitors. Low-risk populations should avoid crowded environments. Employers are allowed to resume unrestricted staffing. Large venues can continue to operate with social distancing and sanitization measures, and bars and restaurants are allowed to increase their standing room capacity. Once this phase is complete, the nation is considered officially reopened, and things can resume as normal. However, the reopening process depends heavily on people adhering to public health guidelines, and travel among neighboring states in different phases of reopening can easily seed new outbreaks. In addition, the White House guidelines are only "strongly encouraged," so it is ultimately up to states to make decisions on the reopening process.[16]

Does reopening mean that I can relax a little with wearing masks and social distancing?

As communities make progress with reopening, people must continue taking precautions to prevent new outbreaks of COVID-19. This means that wearing masks and social distancing are still necessary. Becoming complacent about wearing masks and social distancing is a sure way to amplify and sustain the spread of SARS-CoV-2. Constant vigilance is hard, but the sooner people adhere to public health guidelines, the sooner the pandemic will become a thing of the past.

References

1. Stock JH. Reopening the coronavirus-closed economy. Hutchins Center Working Paper #60. Harvard University Department of Economics & Harvard Kennedy School. Published May 2020.
2. Tucker H. Coronavirus bankruptcy tracker: These major companies are failing amid the shutdown. Forbes. https://www.forbes.com/sites/hanktucker/2020/05/03/coronavirus-bankruptcy-tracker-these-major-companies-are-failing-amid-the-shutdown/#351e1a9a3425. Published 2020. Accessed July 21, 2020.
3. Humphries J, Neilson C, Ulyssea G. The evolving impacts of COVID-19 on small businesses since the CARES Act. SSRN. 2020; Cowles Foundation Discussion Paper No. 2230.
4. Viner RM, Russell SJ, Croker H, et al. School closure and management practices during coronavirus outbreaks including COVID-19: a rapid systematic review. *The Lancet Child & Adolescent Health*. 2020;4(5):397-404.
5. Mannheim J, Gretsch S, Layden J, Fricchione M. Characteristics of hospitalized pediatric coronavirus disease 2019 cases in Chicago, Illinois, March–April 2020. *J Pediatric Infect Dis Soc*. 2020.

6. Centers for Disease Control and Prevention. Provisional COVID-19 death counts by sex, age, and state. https://data.cdc.gov/NCHS/Provisional-COVID-19-Death-Counts-by-Sex-Age-and-S/9bhg-hcku. Published 2020. Accessed July 21, 2020.

7. Williamson L. Corona Virus: Why reopening French schools is a social emergency. BBC News. https://www.bbc.com/news/world-europe-52769626. Published 2020. Accessed July 21, 2020.

8. Patch W. Impact of coronavirus on students' academic progress and college plans – Niche. Niche.com. https://www.niche.com/about/enrollment-insights/impact-of-coronavirus-on-students-academic-progress-and-college-plans/#hssenior. Published 2020. Accessed July 21, 2020.

9. Preskorn SH. The 5% of the population at high risk for severe COVID-19 infection is identifiable and needs to be taken into account when reopening the economy. *J Psychiatr Pract.* 2020;26(3):219–227.

10. Berezow A. Coronavirus: COVID deaths in U.S. by age, race. American Council on Science and Health. https://www.acsh.org/news/2020/06/23/coronavirus-covid-deaths-us-age-race-14863. Published June 25, 2020. Accessed August 8, 2020.

11. Reeves M, Carlsson-Szlezak P, Whitaker K, Abraham M. Sensing and shaping the post-COVID era. BCG Henderson Institute. April 2020.

12. Taylor R. Pros and cons of online learning – a faculty perspective. *Journal of European Industrial Training.* 2002;26(1):24-37.

13. Patch W. Impact of coronavirus on students' academic progress and college plans – Niche. Niche.com. https://www.niche.com/about/enrollment-insights/impact-of-coronavirus-on-students-academic-progress-and-college-plans/#college. Published 2020. Accessed July 22, 2020.

14. Coronavirus cancellations: Admissions testing and college updates. IvyWise. https://www.ivywise.com/blog/corona-virus-cancellations-college-visits-and-admissions-testing/. Published 2020. Accessed July 22, 2020.

15. Müller L-M, Goldenberg G. Education in times of crisis: The potential implications of school closures for teachers and students. Chartered College of Teaching. https://chartered.college/2020/05/07/chartered-college-publishes-report-into-potential-implications-of-school-closures-and-global-approaches-to-education/. Published May 7, 2020. Accessed June 4, 2020.

16. The White House. Opening up America again. https://www.whitehouse.gov/openingamerica/. Published April 2020. Accessed June 4, 2020.

SANITY

How can I reduce the stress from everything that is happening?

Living in the COVID-19 era comes with many emotional challenges: the fear of becoming infected, the stress of financial insecurity, and isolation from loved ones are just a few of these issues. In John Reich's discussion of resilience in natural disasters, Mr. Reich states there are three core principles to coping with natural disasters—the three "3 Cs" of coherence, control, and connectedness. Coherence means understanding more about what is causing the stress—in this case, the pandemic. Improving understanding of COVID-19 is one of the purposes of this book. The second "C," control, refers to individuals having a sense of control over their lives. Due to COVID-19, many people feel they have lost control or had their daily routines halted. When people have a sense of control over their lives, they tend to be happier and less stressed. Lastly, connectedness is relatively self-explanatory, but possibly the most difficult "C" to achieve during these socially distanced times. Fortunately, we live in an era of technology which allows us to communicate with one another. Below are some examples of ways to address the "3 Cs"[2]:

- **Coherence:**
  -Read a book about COVID-19
  -Keep up to date on COVID-19 cases in your area
  -Learn about historic pandemics and how we managed them
  -Learn how to read scientific and research papers
  -Learn the best ways to protect yourself and your family
  -Practice identifying misinformation

- **Control:**
  -Establish a new routine
  -Stay healthy with diet and exercise
  -Practice self-improvement by learning a new skill or language
  -Organize your home and schedule

- **Connectedness:**
  -Hold intentional conversations over the phone or video chat
  -Play games over group video chats
  -Host small in-person social groups outdoors

Aside from the "3 Cs," it is a good habit to limit exposure to social media and news. While it is important to stay informed, these are often sources of negativity that create user engagement through outrage and negative feelings. Setting a time limit on engaging with social media—for example, 30 minutes daily—can help reduce exposure to negative and emotionally draining topics.

How can I keep my kids busy during quarantine?

It is often tempting to preoccupy children with video games and television so that you can focus on your own work during the pandemic. However, this is not the most productive way to use children's time, and it is not ideal for their health. The Child Mind Institute (CMI) provides several tips on productively occupying your child's time.

While the CMI does not entirely condemn the use of technology to occupy kids' time, it is probably best to keep screen time low when possible. The CMI suggests setting up a routine for your child as a way to promote positive habits.[3] Below are two lists of potential activities for your child outside of watching television and playing video games. One list is geared toward independent activities, while the other list suggests activities that can be done together. Of course, many of these activities will depend on your child's age and level of development.

- **Activities to do Alone:**
  -Read
  -Study or do schoolwork
  -Draw, paint, or craft
  -Play with toys like Legos or puzzles that require focus and time
  -Chores and housework

- **Activities to do Together:**
  -Exercise

  -Cook or bake

  -Science experiments (there are plenty of safe and fun science experiments to do with your children!)

  -Play! (hide and seek, build a cushion fort, board games, design a scavenger hunt)

  -Craft

  -Make a time capsule

  -Fix something

  -Home improvement projects

  -Start a family garden

  -Outdoor adventures and hiking

What systems are in place to prevent another pandemic?

Novel viruses with pandemic potential often arise when animal viruses gain the ability to infect humans. Sometimes this produces an extremely contagious virus, as was the case with SARS-CoV-2 when the virus transferred from bats to humans. The sooner the first cross-species infection is identified, the sooner governments can respond to the threat of the virus. Currently, these viral events are monitored through reporting systems like the Global Public Health Intelligence Network (GPHIN).

The GPHIN is an automated web-based scanning system created by Health Canada and the World Health Organization. It scans over 20,000 online news reports daily in nine languages, searching for connections to possible future outbreaks. GPHIN played a role in the initial reporting of the SARS outbreak and monitored the Ebola outbreaks.[4] These reports picked up by GPHIN allowed governments to respond to the SARS outbreak on an international scale. The reporting system quickly notified officials, reported new cases, and helped with tracking sources of infection, which ultimately led to effective quarantining of individuals and regulation of international travel.

Along with GPHIN, we will need to respond to future infectious diseases with pandemic potential more aggressively. This will require greater efforts in isolating infected people, contact tracing, and identifying the pathogen of interest. We will also need to ensure the supply chain of necessary equipment—including personal protective equipment (PPE), diagnostic tests and reagents, and medicine—is capable of handling a surge in demand. Most important of all, countries need to collaborate and communicate with one another to prevent the spread of novel pathogens.[5]

What will the new normal look like?

Society will likely look different after COVID-19. Healthcare, business, and daily life are all likely to change. During the pandemic, telemedicine use skyrocketed: in one New York City healthcare system, telemedicine use for non-urgent complaints increased 40-fold from March 2, 2020 to April 14, 2020.[6] Post-COVID-19, we can expect to see higher usage of telemedicine compared with pre-COVID-19. As medicine will likely turn toward more virtual visits, business is likely to do the same.

We may see a permanent move toward working from home when businesses realize that it is not essential to have employees on-site five days a week. From the consumer end, there has been a large uptick in online shopping. The pandemic has put additional stress on brick-and-mortar retail and department stores, which were already under pressure from online shopping. Physical stores may recover some after the pandemic passes, but we are likely to see a greater percentage of sales move online compared with pre-pandemic times.[7]

From an employment perspective, we may see an increase in manufacturing jobs if manufacturing companies return to the United States. With the pandemic straining supply chains, moving manufacturing of essential supplies domestically could both produce jobs and prevent critical supply shortages in the future.

From an everyday standpoint, people may be more conscientious about social distancing and respecting one another's personal space, either out of fear or a greater appreciation for personal space. COVID-19 will certainly have a lasting impact on our day-to-day lives, and some of these changes will be unpredictable.

How can I help?

The most important thing you can do to help is simply do your part in preventing the spread of SARS-CoV-2: wear a mask in public, wash your hands, social distance, minimize travel, and pay attention to your health. If you are sick, either self-quarantine or seek medical attention.

However, if you would like to help out more and contribute to your community, there are many ways to help in these difficult times. Below are some ways you can help others either directly through action or indirectly through monetary contributions.[8] This is not intended to be an all-encompassing list. If none of these suggestions appeal to you, simply look online for ways you can help locally.

· **Monetary donations:**

-The **Boys and Girls Clubs of America** raises funds to provide food for children nationally.

-**Meals on Wheels** delivers subsidized meals to the elderly.

-**Local food banks** are always in need of nutritious, non-perishable food.

-The **CDC Foundation** helps coordinate assistance in areas of need, supplies PPE, and tracks COVID-19 cases.

-The **Restaurant Workers' Community Foundation** provides financial support to service workers struggling to make a living.

-**Local hospitals** may accept unused PPE.

· **Volunteer Opportunities:**

-Schedule a donation with **the American Red Cross or local blood banks** to help with blood shortages.

-Offer **daycare for essential workers**. Many medical staff and other essential workers do not have the option to work from home, and without school and summer programs there are volunteer programs to help with childcare.

-**Deliver groceries to elderly** or other high-risk individuals.

-**Kindness Calls for Seniors** helps elderly people maintain connections and cope with isolation during COVID-19.

Is COVID-19 ever going away?

SARS-CoV-2 and COVID-19 are likely here to stay. Early in the pandemic—and especially before SARS-CoV-2 began spreading outside of China—it might have been possible to contain the virus with strict lockdowns, aggressive contact tracing, and strong adherence to public health guidelines. For example, New Zealand successfully eliminated the virus within its borders for a time, although in early August the virus was reintroduced to the country through an unknown border failure.

However, now that SARS-CoV-2 has spread widely across the planet, it is likely to continue circulating. It will not be the first coronavirus to do so: four other coronaviruses circulate among humans and frequently cause the common cold.[9] Fortunately, over time, respiratory viruses tend to accumulate mutations which make them less dangerous. This is because the only goals of a virus are to multiply and continue infecting new hosts, and viruses that are too deadly—in other words, those that kill their hosts—are more likely to die out than viruses that cause mild disease. Scientists have hypothesized that many of the viruses that cause the common cold started as pandemics.[9] Over time, these viruses became less lethal and people gained immunity against them, making the diseases they cause relatively mild.

In short, the novel coronavirus is not going away, but as more people develop immunity and the virus mutates, COVID-19 may become a less severe disease. However, this is a very slow process that occurs over years, so in the meantime it is important to continue wearing masks and practice social distancing.

References

1. Reich, J. W. Three psychological principles of resilience in natural disasters. *Disaster Prevention and Management: An International Journal.* 2006; 15(5), 793-798.

2. Polizzi C, Lynn SJ, Perry A. Stress and coping in the time of COVID-19: Pathways to resilience and recovery. *Clinical Neuropsychiatry.* 2020;17(2):59-62.

3. Sheldon-Dean H. Screen time during the coronavirus crisis. Child Mind Institute. https://childmind.org/article/screen-time-during-the-coronavirus-crisis/. Published May 27, 2020. Accessed August 8, 2020.

4. Dion M, Abdel-Malik P, Mawudeku A. Big data and the global public health intelligence network (GPHIN). *Can Commun Dis Rep.* 2015;41(9):209–214. Published 2015 Sep 3.

5. Triggle CR, Bansal D, Farag EABA, Ding H, Sultan AA. COVID-19: Learning from lessons to guide treatment and prevention interventions. *mSphere.* 2020;5(3):e00317-20. Published 2020 May 13.

6. Mann DM, Chen J, Chunara R, Testa PA, Nov O. COVID-19 transforms health care through telemedicine: evidence from the field [published online ahead of print, 2020 Apr 23]. *J Am Med Inform Assoc.* 2020.

7. Taherian S. The New World: How the world will be different after COVID-19. *Forbes.* https://www.forbes.com/sites/suzytaherian/2020/04/07/the-new-world-how-the-world-will-be-different-

after-covid-19/#329d01555d15. Published April 7, 2020. Accessed June 12, 2020.

8. Vongkiatkajorn K, Daily L. How you can help during the coronavirus outbreak. *The Washington Post.* https://www.washingtonpost.com/nation/2020/03/21/how-you-can-help-during-coronavirus/?arc404=true. Published April 6, 2020. Accessed June 10, 2020.

9. Zhang S. The coronavirus is never going away. *The Atlantic.* https://www.theatlantic.com/health/archive/2020/08/coronavirus-will-never-go-away/614860/. Published August 4, 2020. Accessed August 16, 2020.

ABOUT THE AUTHORS

Dr. Steven R. Feldman is a Professor of Dermatology, Pathology, Social Sciences & Health Policy, and Molecular Medicine & Translational Science at the Wake Forest School of Medicine. Dr. Feldman's chief clinical interest is psoriasis—a chronic, physically and psychosocially disabling condition—and he was among the first authors to publish on the impact of COVID-19 on the treatment of psoriasis patients. He serves on the COVID-19 Task Force of the National Psoriasis Foundation and is an author of the "Coronavirus disease 2019 (COVID-19): Cutaneous manifestations and issues related to dermatologic care" chapter of *UpToDate*. He has given more than 700 invited lectures to medical groups and organizations around the world, including the Pan Arab Dermatology Meeting held in Riyadh, Saudi Arabia; the Iranian Dermatology Society meeting in Tehran, Iran; and the Pan Asian Dermatology Meeting held in Seoul, South Korea. His research has been published in over 1,000 Medline reference articles. Dr. Feldman also serves as the editor of the *Journal of Dermatological Treatment* and the *Journal of Dermatology and Dermatological Surgery* and as chief medical editor of *The Dermatologist*.

Veronica Emmerich is a medical student at the Wake Forest School of Medicine. Before medicine, she studied political science at the University of California, Santa Barbara and biochemistry at North Carolina State University. While studying biochemistry, she worked in a virology lab studying viruses that cause infectious diseases such as Zika, Chikungunya, and Dengue fever.